Understanding Pediatric Heart Sounds

Understanding Pediatric Heart Sounds

second edition

Steven Lehrer, MD
The Mount Sinai School of Medicine
New York, New York

Saunders
An Imprint of Elsevier Science
Philadelphia   London   New York   St. Louis   Sydney   Toronto

SAUNDERS
An Imprint of Elsevier Science

11830 Westline Industrial Drive
St. Louis, Missouri 63146

Understanding Pediatric Heart Sounds   ISBN 1468138030
Copyright © 2003, Elsevier Science (USA). All rights reserved.   9781468138030

NOTICE

Health care is an ever-changing field. Standard safety precautions must be followed, but as new research and clinical experience broaden our knowledge, changes in treatment and drug therapy may become necessary or appropriate. Readers are advised to check the most current product information provided by the manufacturer of each drug to be administered to verify the recommended dose, the method and duration of administration, and contraindications. It is the responsibility of the licensed health care provider, relying on experience and knowledge of the patient, to determine dosages and the best treatment for each individual patient. Neither the publisher nor the editor assumes any liability for any injury and/or damage to persons or property arising from this publication.

Previous edition copyrighted 1992
Library of Congress Cataloging-in-Publication Data
Lehrer, Steven.
   Understanding pediatric heart sounds / Steven Lehrer.—2nd ed.
     p. ; cm.
   Includes bibliographical references and index.
   ISBN 0-7216-9646-5
    1. Pediatric cardiology—Diagnosis. 2. Heart—Sounds. I. Title.
    [DNLM: 1. Heart Valve Diseases—Child. 2. Heart Valve Diseases—Infant. 3. Heart Auscultation—Child. 4. Heart Auscultation—Infant. 5. Heart Sounds—Child. 6. Heart Sounds—Infant. WG 260 L524u 2003]
   RJ423 .L44 2003
   618.92¢1207544—dc21
                            2002026834

Vice President and Publishing Director: Sally Schrefer
Acquisitions Editor: Loren Wilson
Developmental Editor: Nancy L. O'Brien
Publishing Services Manager: John Rogers
Project Manager: Doug Turner
Designer: Kathi Gosche
Cover Art: Kathi Gosche

RT/MVY

Printed in the United States of America.
Last digit is the print number: 9   8   7   6   5   4   3   2   1

Preface

In 1896, Dr. Thomas Morgan Rotch, Professor of Diseases of Children at Harvard Medical School, published a textbook of pediatrics. As Dr. Alexander Nadas noted, only seven of 1100 pages dealt with congenital disease of the heart.

"It is usually possible to make a diagnosis of congenital heart disease," wrote Dr. Rotch, but "a diagnosis of the especial lesion is, as a rule, impossible." Indeed, the precise diagnosis was only of academic interest, because so little could be done for the patient. Dr. Rotch did mention that "the administration of digitalis in small doses with the utmost caution" was sometimes useful, but treatment was "essentially hygienic and symptomatic."

Another Harvard pediatrician, Professor John Lovett Morse, wrote a new pediatrics textbook in 1926. Morse devoted 40 pages to heart disease, of which less than five dealt with congenital abnormalities.

Even the development of the x-ray had little impact on the diagnosis and treatment of congenital heart disease. "The Roentgen ray, which theoretically ought to be of considerable assistance in the diagnosis of special lesions, is practically of little assistance even in the hands of an expert," wrote Dr. Morse. "Fortunately the diagnosis of the exact lesion is not of great importance in either prognosis or treatment. There is no curative treatment [and] nothing which will either diminish the deformities or favor the closure of abnormal openings. The treatment must, therefore, be hygienic and symptomatic."

The Blalock-Taussig shunt operation and the subsequent development of cardiovascular surgery revolutionized the treatment of heart disease in children. Heart deformities and abnormal openings could frequently be repaired, though precise diagnosis was a problem. The only certain diagnostic method was cardiac catheterization, an invasive technique. However, a physician skilled with a stethoscope could often make a correct diagnosis at the bedside.

In the last decade, the perfection of echocardiography, Doppler ultrasonography, and magnetic resonance imaging has made possible the accurate diagnosis of many structural heart abnormalities by noninvasive methods. As a result, very few students receive the detailed instruction in the use of a stethoscope that would allow them to diagnose most pediatric heart problems.

Not all children are examined in a hospital setting. A stethoscope is still the best diagnostic tool when a child is examined at home, in school, or for the first time in the clinic. This book provides the information a caregiver needs to become proficient at pediatric cardiac auscultation.

Steven Lehrer
New York City

Acknowledgments

I wish to thank the following colleagues for their assistance: Dr. Eva Botstein Griepp, who reviewed both the manuscript and the audio CD; Dr. Jerome Liebman and Dr. C. K. Lowe, who reviewed the manuscript; Ms. Katherine Pitcoff, who edited the manuscript; and Mr. Mark Warner, who helped to make the audio CD.

S_1, S_2, systolic ejection sound, midsystolic click, murmurs of mitral regurgitation, tricuspid regurgitation, aortic stenosis, aortic regurgitation, patent ductus arteriosus, atrial septal defect, and whoop are from **Physical Examination of the Heart and Circulation, Cardiac Auscultation** (1984), by Joseph K. Perloff and Mark E. Silverman and are reproduced by kind permission of the American College of Cardiology.

Still's murmur, cervical venous hum, and murmur of ventricular septal defect are from **The Guide to Heart Sounds: Normal and Abnormal** (1988), by Donald W. Novey, Marcia Pencak, and John M. Stang. These sounds were produced by the Cardionics Heart Sound Simulator, Cardionics, Inc., Houston, Texas. They are reproduced by kind permission of Dr. Novey, Mr. Keith Johnson of Cardionics, and CRC Press, Inc., Boca Raton, Florida.

S_3, S_4, quadruple rhythm, and summation gallop are from **Understanding Heart Sounds and Murmurs**, 3rd edition (2001), by Ara G. Tilkian and Mary Boudreau Conover, WB Saunders Company, Philadelphia, and were also produced on the Cardionics Heart Sound Simulator, Cardionics, Inc., Houston, Texas.

First pericardial friction rub was lent by Dr. W. Proctor Harvey. Second pericardial friction rub is from **Essentials of Bedside Cardiology** (1988), by Jules Constant, Little Brown, Boston, and is reproduced by kind permission of Dr. Constant and the publisher.

Murmur of Blalock-Taussig shunt was produced with the Heart Sounds Tutor, Wolff Industries, San Marino, California, and is reproduced by permission.

Contents

Chapter **10**
General Characteristics of Murmurs 119

Chapter **11**
Systolic Murmurs 125

Chapter **12**
Diastolic Murmurs   161

Chapter **13**

Continuous Murmurs 173

Chapter **14**

Surgically Created Shunts and Prosthetic Valves 185

Chapter **15**
Complex Anomalies 193

Contents of Audio CD

Track 1. First and second heart sounds, S_1 and S_2
Track 2. Third heart sound, S_3
Track 3. Fourth heart sound, S_4
Track 4. Quadruple rhythm
Track 5. Summation gallop
Track 6. Systolic ejection sound
Track 7. Midsystolic click
Track 8. Still's murmur
Track 9. Murmur of mitral regurgitation
Track 10. Murmur of tricuspid regurgitation
Track 11. Murmur of aortic stenosis
Track 12. Murmur of pulmonic stenosis
Track 13. Murmur of aortic regurgitation
Track 14. Murmur of patent ductus arteriosus
Track 15. Cervical venous hum
Track 16. Murmur of a Blalock-Taussig shunt
Track 17. Murmur of ventricular septal defect
Track 18. Murmur of atrial septal defect
Track 19. Late systolic whoop
Track 20. Pericardial friction rub

Complete contents of audio CD may be downloaded from
http://stevenlehrer.com/heart.htm
or heard at
http://www.youtube.com/watch?v=lp8gUJQvsSs

Chapter 1

The Heart as a Pump

The heart, which functions as a pump to push blood through the vascular system, actually consists of two pumps: a right heart that pumps blood through the lungs, and a left heart that pumps blood through the peripheral organs and tissues. Each of these units is made up of two chambers, an **atrium** and a **ventricle.**

A system of valves controls the flow of blood through these pumps. The atria are separated from the ventricles by the atrioventricular (AV) valves (the tricuspid and mitral valves). The aorta and pulmonary arteries are separated from the ventricles by the semilunar valves (the aortic and pulmonic valves) (discussed later).

The atrium is a weak pump. Although it helps to move blood, the atrium serves principally as an entrance to the ventricle. The ventricle supplies the energy necessary to force blood through the pulmonary and systemic circulations. Figure 1-1 illustrates the structure of the heart and the direction of the blood flow within it. Note the two primer pumps (the atria) and the two power pumps (the ventricles).

Because the right and left sides of the heart have different functions, the right and left ventricles are not structurally identical. The right ventricle (supplying the pulmonary circulation) pumps against a much lower resistance and is thinner walled than the left ventricle. Interestingly, the right atrium alone is capable of pumping blood through the pulmonary circulation and does so postoperatively in children who have undergone the Fontan procedure for tricuspid atresia (see Chapter 15).

THE CARDIAC CYCLE
Electrical Events in the Cardiac Cycle

The cardiac cycle is the interval from the end of one contraction of the heart to the end of the next. Each cycle is triggered by the spontaneous generation of an action potential in the sinoatrial (SA) node, found in the anterior wall of the right atrium near the opening of the superior vena cava (Figure 1-2). From the SA node the action potential follows a path through both atria to

1

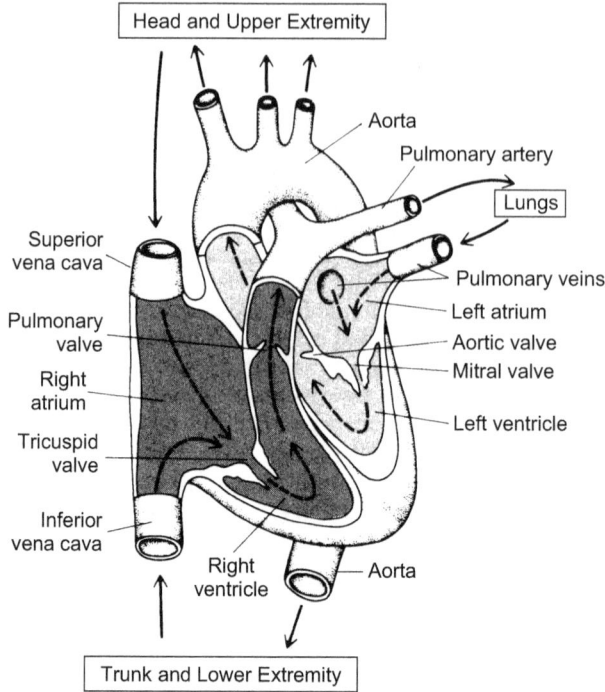

Figure 1-1. Structure of the heart and course of blood flow through the heart chambers. (From Guyton AC, Hall JE: **Textbook of medical physiology,** ed 10, Philadelphia, 2000, WB Saunders.)

the AV node, to the AV bundle, and then into the ventricles. Because of the structure of the conducting system, the action potential is delayed 0.10 second between the atria and the ventricles. This delay allows the atria to contract before the ventricles, delivering blood to the ventricles before their very forceful contraction.

The Purkinje fibers, which lead from the AV node through the AV bundle and into the ventricles, conduct the action potential throughout the entire ventricular system. Once past the AV bundle, the fibers divide almost immediately into the left and right bundle branches, which spread downward toward the apex of the ventricles. The fibers further divide into small branches, which extend around each ventricular chamber and back toward the base of the heart. The Purkinje fibers penetrate the muscle mass to end on muscle fibers.

Mechanical Events in the Cardiac Cycle

The cardiac cycle is composed of a period of ventricular contraction, called **systole,** followed by a period of ventricular relaxation, called **diastole**. Figure

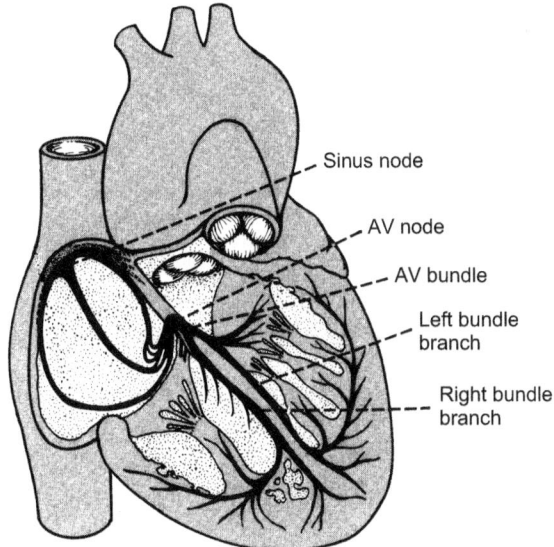

Figure 1-2. The sinus node and the Purkinje system of the heart, showing also the AV node and the ventricular bundle branches. (From Guyton AC, Hall JE: **Textbook of medical physiology,** ed 10, Philadelphia, 2000, WB Saunders.)

1-3 illustrates the events occurring during these periods. The upper three curves demonstrate pressure changes in the aorta, the left ventricle, and the left atrium, and the fourth curve shows changes in ventricular volume. The fifth and sixth lines are the **electrocardiogram** (ECG) and **phonocardiogram** (a recording of the sounds made by the heart as it pumps), respectively.

The ECG shows the P, Q, R, S, and T waves, electrical impulses generated by the heart and recorded by the electrocardiograph from the surface of the body. The **P wave** results from the spread of depolarization through the atria, followed by atrial contraction, which causes a slight elevation in the atrial pressure curve immediately after the P wave.

Shortly after the beginning of the P wave, the **QRS complex** appears. The QRS complex results from ventricular depolarization. The interval between the beginning of the P wave and the QRS complex is called the **P-R interval.** In adults, the average P-R interval is 0.16 second. In children, the **P-R interval** varies with age and heart rate (Table 1-1). Ventricular depolarization initiates ventricular contraction and produces a ventricular pressure rise (see Figure 1-3). The QRS complex always occurs just before the beginning of ventricular systole.

Following the QRS complex, the **T wave** appears. This wave is the result of ventricular repolarization accompanied by relaxation of the ventricular muscle fibers. The T wave is seen just before the end of ventricular contraction.

Blood flows continually into the atria from the great veins (the superior vena cava, the inferior vena cava, and the pulmonary veins). Normally, 70% of this blood passes directly through the atria into the ventricles before atrial

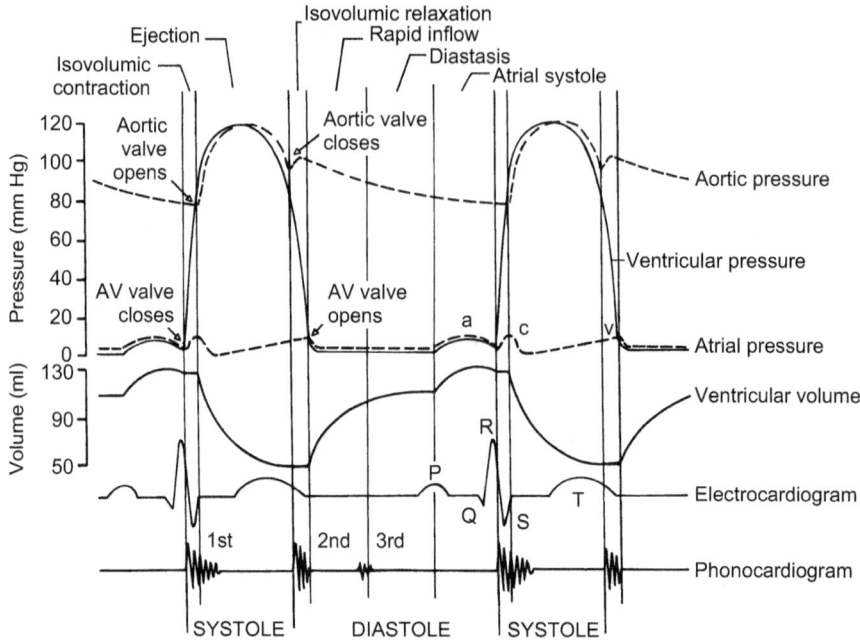

Figure 1-3. The events of the cardiac cycle, showing changes in left atrial pressure, left ventricular pressure, aortic pressure, ventricular volume, the electrocardiogram, and the phonocardiogram. (From Guyton AC, Hall JE: **Textbook of medical physiology,** ed 10, Philadelphia, 2000, WB Saunders.)

TABLE 1–1. Maximal P-R Intervals in Seconds at Different Age Levels and Varying Heart Rates

Age	Rate					
	< 71	71-90	91-110	111-130	131-150	> 150
<1 month			0.11	0.11	0.11	0.11
1–9 months			0.14	0.13	0.12	0.11
10–24 months			0.15	0.14	0.14	0.10
3–5 years		0.16	0.16	0.16	0.13	
6–13 years	0.18	0.18	0.16	0.16		

From Alimurung MM, Massell BF: The normal P-R interval in infants and children, **Circulation** 13:257, 1956.

contraction. An additional 20% to 30% of ventricular filling results from atrial contraction. Even without atrial contraction, the heart can continue to function adequately under normal resting conditions, because the ventricles are capable of pumping three to four times more blood than the body requires.

There are three major fluctuations in the atrial pressure curve during the cardiac cycle—the A, C, and V waves (see Figure 1-3). The **A wave** results from atrial contraction. The right atrial pressure increases 4 to 6 mm Hg, and the left atrial pressure increases 7 to 8 mm Hg. The **C wave** appears when ventricular contraction begins and is caused by (1) the slight backflow of blood into the atria and (2) the bulging of the atrioventricular valves backward into the atria because of rising ventricular pressure. The **V wave** is seen near the end of ventricular contraction and is caused by the gradual accumulation of blood in the atria while the AV valves are closed during ventricular contraction. When the AV valves open at the end of ventricular contraction, blood courses rapidly into the ventricles and the V wave vanishes.

VENTRICULAR FUNCTION
Diastolic Ventricular Filling

Because the AV valves are closed during ventricular contraction, a large quantity of blood accumulates in the atria. At the end of ven-tricular systole, intraventricular pressure falls to its low diastolic value, and the relatively high atrial pressure pushes the AV valves open, permitting a rapid flow of blood into the ventricles. This phase of **rapid ventricular filling** is seen as a rise in the ventricular volume curve (see Figure 1-3). Note that atrial and ventricular pressures are almost equal at this time because the AV valve orifices are large and offer practically no resistance to blood flow. This phase of rapid filling occupies the first third of diastole.

Relatively little blood enters the ventricles during the middle third of diastole. The blood has emptied into the atria from the great veins and flows directly into the ventricles. This period when blood flow is almost at a standstill is called **diastasis**. During the last third of diastole, the atria contract. As mentioned, 20% to 30% of ventricular filling is due to atrial contraction.

Systolic Ventricular Emptying

Isovolumic (Isometric) Contraction
When ventricular contraction commences, there is a sharp ventricular pressure rise (see Figure 1-3), forcing the AV valves to close. It takes 0.02 to 0.03 second for the ventricle to develop sufficient pressure to force the semilunar valves open; that is, to exceed the pressures in the aorta and pulmonary artery. During this isovolumic phase, the ventricles are contract-ing but not emptying.

Ejection Phase
When the semilunar valves are pushed open, blood rushes out of the ventricles. About 70% of the blood in the ventricles is emptied during

the first third of the ejection phase, called the **period of rapid ejection**. The final 30% is emptied in the last two thirds of the ejection phase, called the **period of slow ejection**.

During the period of slow ejection, ventricular pressure falls slightly below aortic pressure, even though some blood is still flowing out of the left ventricle. The pressure fall occurs because the outflowing blood has acquired momentum, the kinetic energy of which is manifested as aortic pressure.

The blood flow sequence just described is illustrated in Figure 1-4. In this series of diagrams, a computer model has been used to reveal details of fluid motion not visible in human studies or animal experiments.

Isovolumic (Isometric) Relaxation

At the end of systole, ventricular relaxation commences suddenly, and intraventricular pressure falls rapidly. In the distended large arteries, heightened pressures abruptly force blood back toward the ventricles, snapping the aortic and pulmonic valves shut. The ventricular muscle relaxes for 0.03 to 0.06 second, although the ventricular volume remains constant. This interval is called the **phase of isovolumic (isometric) relaxation**. When the intraventricular pressures reach their low diastolic levels, the AV valves open and begin a new pumping cycle.

The Frank-Starling Law

What causes blood to flow into the heart during diastole? Since early in this century, the accepted mechanism of the heart's pumping function has been based on the work of two investigators, Otto Frank and Ernest H. Starling. The Frank-Starling law basically states that the more the heart is filled during diastole, the greater the quantity of blood pumped into the aorta; this law explains how the heart can adapt, from moment to moment, to widely varying influxes of blood.

Until recently, cardiologists assumed that once systolic contraction was complete, diastolic filling was a completely passive process. However, studies by Robinson and colleagues (1986) suggest that filling is an active process. Some energy from each contraction is stored within the muscle, causing the heart to function as a suction pump during diastole. The suction power is amplified by the motion of the heart within the chest. This action can be compared to a machine gun, which uses the force generated by the firing of one cartridge to provide the energy needed to load the next shot.

THE CARDIAC VALVES AND PAPILLARY MUSCLES

The AV valves (the **tricuspid** and **mitral valves**) separate the atria from the ventricles and keep blood from flowing backward from the ventricles into

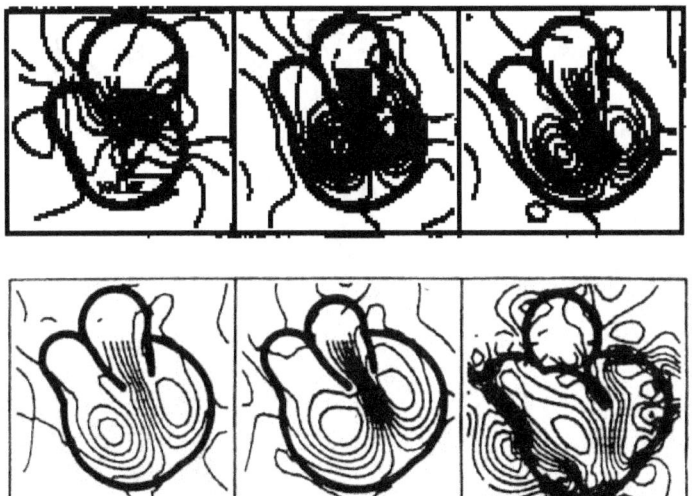

Figure 1-4. A computer model of blood flow through the heart. Note the two chambers representing the left atrium and the left ventricle, separated by the mitral valve. As the left atrium contracts, blood flows downward. Whirling vortices form in the left ventricle (the lower chamber), expanding the heart walls. Pumping motion begins and the mitral valve closes. In this model, the heart is considered to be immersed in a beaker of fluid, and vortices form outside as well as inside the chambers. Engineers and physiologists are now using this model to test new designs for artificial heart valves. (From McQueen DM, Peskin CS, Yellin EL: Fluid dynamics of the mitral valve: physiological aspects of a mathematical model, **Am J Physiol** 242:H1095-H1110, 1982.)

the atria during systole. The **semilunar valves** (the **aortic** and **pulmonic valves**) keep blood from flowing backward from the aorta and pulmonary arteries into the ventricles during diastole. The four valves open and close passively (Figures 1-5 and 1-6). In other words, they open when forced forward and close when forced backward. The thin, filmy AV valves need very little backflow to be forced closed. The thicker semilunar valves need a few milliseconds of stronger backflow to be closed.

The papillary muscles are connected to the leaflets of the AV valves by chordae tendineae (see Figure 1-5). The papillary muscles contract with the ventricles, pulling the leaflets inward toward the ventricular wall to prevent their bulging into the atria during systole. Should a papillary muscle rupture or become paralyzed, the leaflet bulges far backward, resulting in a serious leak and sometimes heart failure.

The elevated arterial pressure at the end of systole snaps the semilunar valves shut. In contrast, the thinner AV valves close more gradually. Furthermore, blood is forced more quickly through the semilunar valves than through the considerably larger AV valves. The rapid closure and increased blood flow cause the semilunar valves to sustain more wear than the

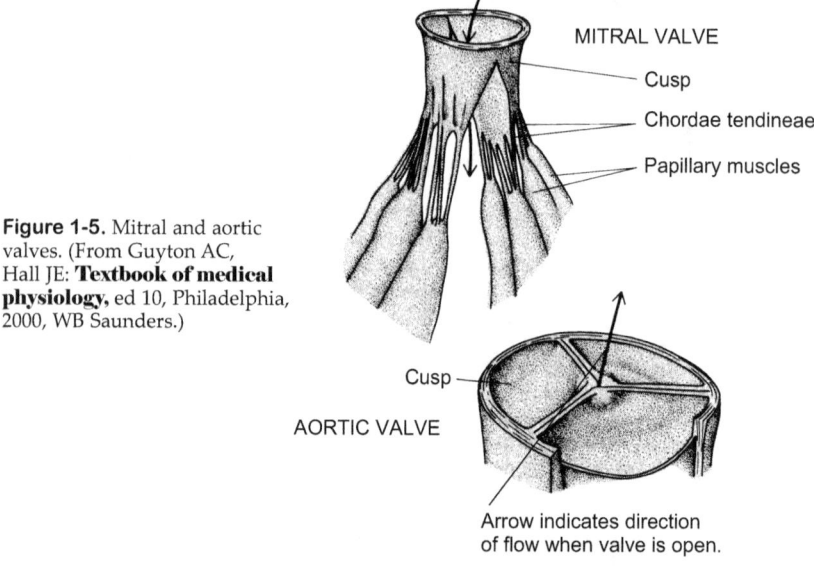

Figure 1-5. Mitral and aortic valves. (From Guyton AC, Hall JE: **Textbook of medical physiology,** ed 10, Philadelphia, 2000, WB Saunders.)

MITRAL VALVE

— Cusp

— Chordae tendineae

— Papillary muscles

Cusp

AORTIC VALVE

Arrow indicates direction of flow when valve is open.

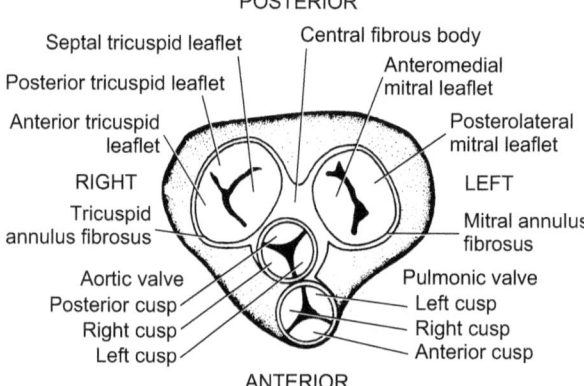

POSTERIOR

Septal tricuspid leaflet

Posterior tricuspid leaflet

Anterior tricuspid leaflet

RIGHT

Tricuspid annulus fibrosus

Aortic valve
Posterior cusp
Right cusp
Left cusp

Central fibrous body

Anteromedial mitral leaflet

Posterolateral mitral leaflet

LEFT

Mitral annulus fibrosus

Pulmonic valve
Left cusp
Right cusp
Anterior cusp

ANTERIOR

Figure 1-6. Schematic anterosuperior view of the heart with the atria removed. The components of the fibrous skeleton and the orientation of the leaflets of each valve are demonstrated. The fibrous skeleton provides a firm anchorage for the attachments of the atrial and ventricular musculatures as well as the valvular tissue. (From Schant RC, Silverman ME: Anatomy of the heart. In Hurst JW, Logue RB, Rackley CE et al, editors: **The heart,** ed 6, New York, 1986, McGraw-Hill.)

AV valves (Figure 1-7).

Considered as a feat of engineering, the heart valves are remarkable. They must function flawlessly two or three billion times over the course of a human lifetime. In addition, their perfectly adapted structure allows the

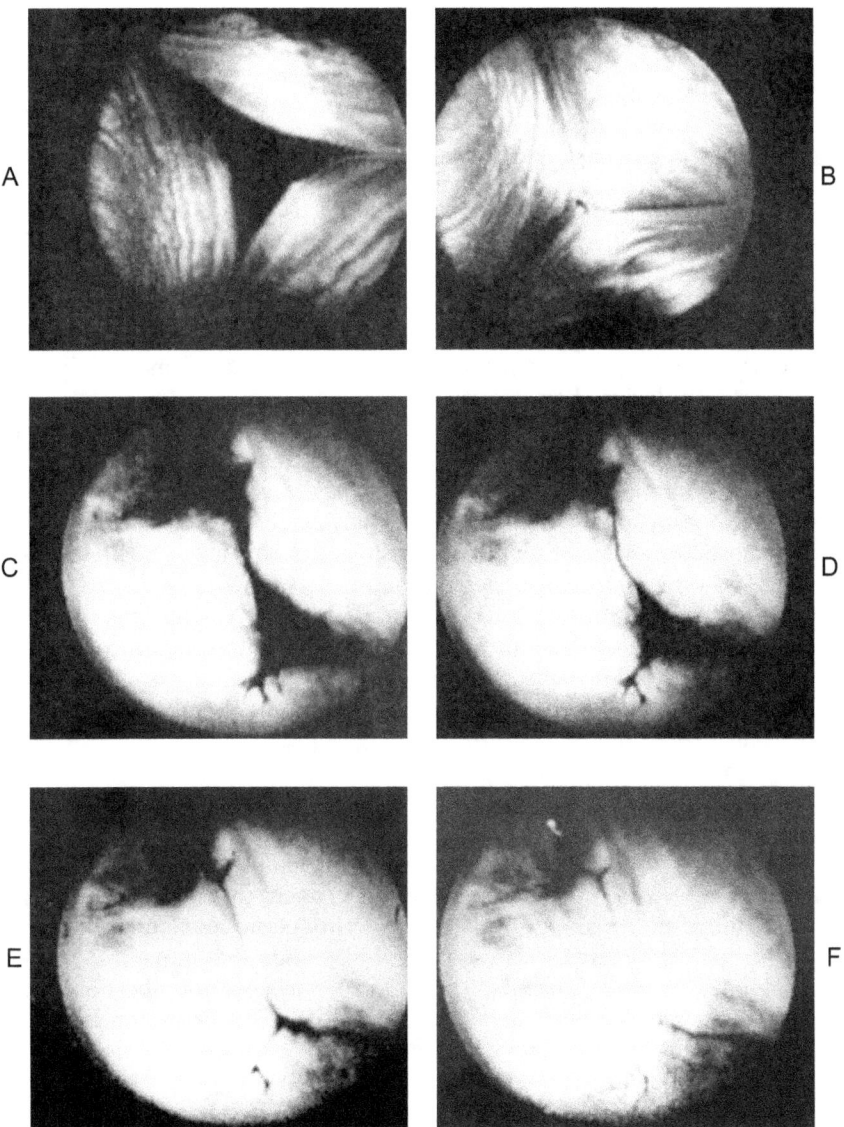

Figure 1-7. Functioning heart valves: **A** and **B** show successive frames from a motion picture (made at the speed of 24 frames per second) of the closing of the pulmonic valve in an isolated beef heart. **C** to **F** show a comparable series in the closure of the tricuspid valve in the same heart. The tricuspid valve took about twice as long to close and closed first at the middle. Faster closure of the arterial valves may be partly responsible for the fact that the second heart sound is usually shorter, with more high-frequency components than the first. (From film PMF 5162 made by the Armed Forces Institute of Pathology. In McKusick VA: **Cardiovascular sound in health and disease,** Baltimore, 1958, Williams & Wilkins.)

passage of blood without damage or clotting. Engineers have not done nearly so well, although artificial heart valves, made of metal, plastic, or pyrolytic carbon, are now in widespread use (see Chapter 14).

THE AORTIC PRESSURE CURVE

As the ventricle contracts, ventricular pressure rises quickly until the aortic valve opens. Thereafter, ventricular pressure increases less, because blood is flowing out of the ventricle into the aorta (see Figure 1-3). As blood flows into the arteries, it distends their walls, and the pressure within them rises. At the end of systole, when the left ventricle ceases to pump blood and the aortic valve closes, elastic recoil of the arteries maintains an elevated pressure, even during diastole.

When the aortic valve shuts, an incisura (or notch) is seen in the aortic pressure curve (see Figure 1-3). The incisura results from the short interval of backflow immediately before the valve closes, followed by sudden cessation of the backflow. Closure of the aortic valve is followed by a slow fall in aortic pressure throughout diastole (to 80 mm Hg in the adult), because blood within the distended arteries is flowing outward to the peripheral vessels and veins. The normal aortic blood pressure values of 120 mm Hg systolic and 80 mm Hg diastolic are adult averages. In children these pressures are lower and vary with age. The pulmonary artery pressure curve resembles that of the aorta, except that pulmonic pressures are only about one sixth as high.

HEART SOUNDS AND HEART FUNCTION

The opening of cardiac valves cannot normally be heard through the stethoscope. When the opening is audible, as in mild aortic or pulmonic stenosis, the resulting sound is called an **ejection click** (see Chapter 9).

The closing of cardiac valves produces sounds that move in all directions, known as **heart sounds**. The sound is the result of vibration of the valve leaflets and surrounding fluids. The following discussion is a brief introduction to the generation of heart sounds. The topic is discussed in detail in the following chapters.

When systole begins, the **first heart sound** (S_1) is produced by the closure of the AV (mitral and tricuspid) valves. This sound is low-pitched and relatively long (see Figure 1-3).

The quick closing of the aortic and pulmonic valves generates a shorter, sharper sound, the **second heart sound** (S_2). The sound is shorter because the leaflets of these valves and surrounding fluids vibrate for a comparatively shorter interval.

The **third heart sound** (S_3) is a normal finding in children and young adults. It is caused by the sudden, intrinsic limitation of longitudinal expansion of the ventricular wall. The abrupt jerk produces low-frequency vibrations that constitute the third heart sound.

The **fourth heart sound** (S₄) is produced by vibrations in the expanding ventricles during the second phase of rapid diastolic filling when the atria contract. S₄ is also called an **atrial sound,** an **atrial gallop,** or a **presystolic gallop**.

CIRCULATORY CHANGES AT BIRTH

During fetal life, pulmonary blood flow is about 10% to 15% of combined ventricular output; the lungs are two-thirds filled with fluid; and pulmonary vascular resistance is high because of low blood oxygen content (Po_2). Animal studies have confirmed the relationship of pulmonary vascular resistance and blood oxygen content.

Experiments on pregnant sheep have shown that if the lungs of the fetus are fully expanded without oxygen, pulmonary vascular resistance does not drop normally after birth. If the ewe receives abnormally high amounts of oxygen (hyperbaric oxygen), pulmonary vascular resistance in the fetus drops.

Another factor may also contribute to the low pulmonary blood flow in the fetus. Because there is very little resistance to blood flow through the placenta, almost all pulmonary arterial blood is channeled through the ductus arteriosus (Figure 1-8, A) and into the aorta rather than through the lungs. The blood is oxygenated by the mother in the placenta and does not need to pass through the lungs for oxygenation. Blood flow through the lungs is needed for pulmonary maturation.

When the baby is born, its lungs immediately inflate. The alveoli fill with air, and pulmonary vascular resistance falls abruptly and dramatically (although it does not reach adult levels until 6 to 8 weeks after birth). At the same time, aortic pressure increases because blood flow through the placenta has suddenly stopped. Pulmonary pressure falls, aortic pressure rises, and blood, which had been flowing forward from the pulmonary artery through the ductus arteriosus to the aorta, begins to flow backward, from the aorta through the ductus to the pulmonary artery. These changes occur over several hours.

Before birth, the ductus arteriosus is probably kept open by a prostaglandin, a hormone found within its wall, although the exact mechanism is unknown. Ten to fifteen hours after the birth of a normal, full-term infant, the ductus arteriosus closes, and blood flow through it stops. The trigger for closure may be the postnatal rise in arterial oxygen tension. It is not clear whether oxygen affects the smooth muscle cells of the ductus directly or an additional agent is involved. Sometimes the ductus arteriosus requires several weeks to close completely, and in 1 of every 5500 infants, the ductus never closes. The resulting condition, **patent ductus arteriosus,** is discussed in Chapter 11.

Another circulatory change that takes place at birth is in the atrial septum,

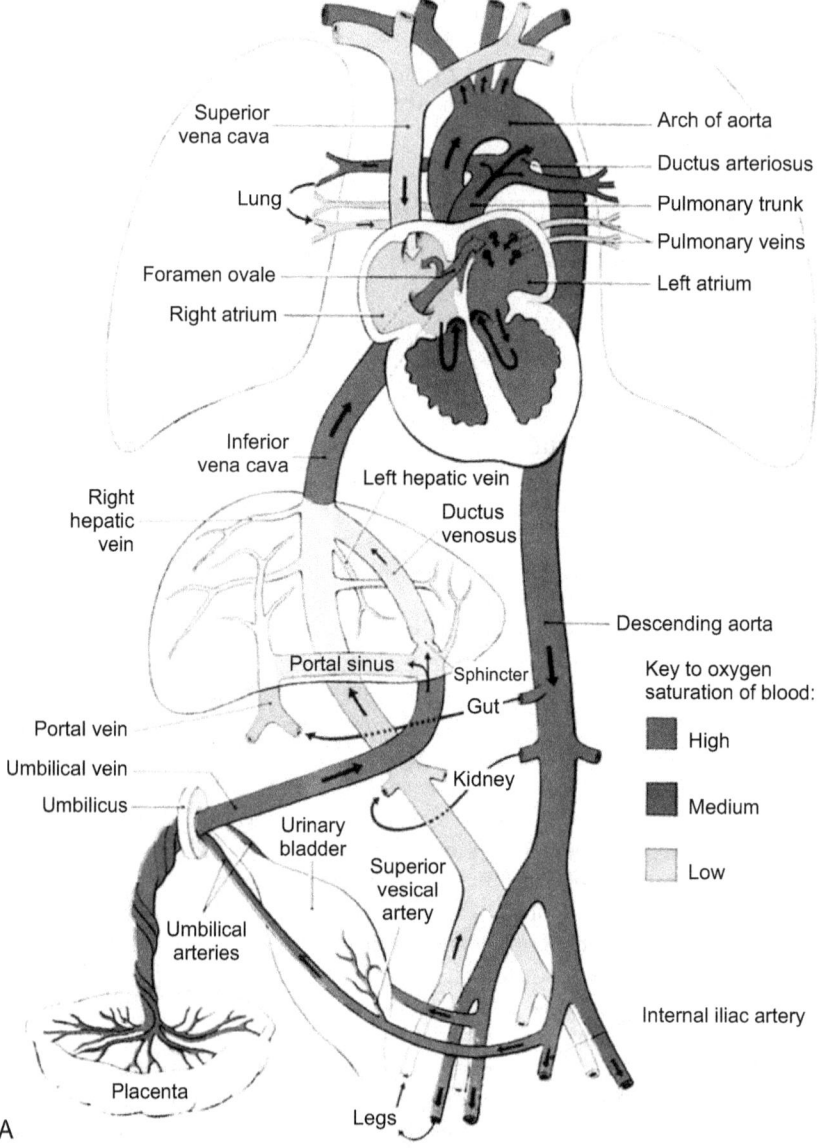

Figure 1-8. A, Simplified scheme of the fetal circulation. The darkened areas indicate the oxygen saturation of the blood, and the arrows show the course of the fetal circulation. The organs are not drawn to scale. Three shunts permit most of the blood to bypass the liver and lungs: (1) the ductus venosus, (2) the foramen ovale, and (3) the ductus arteriosus.

Continued

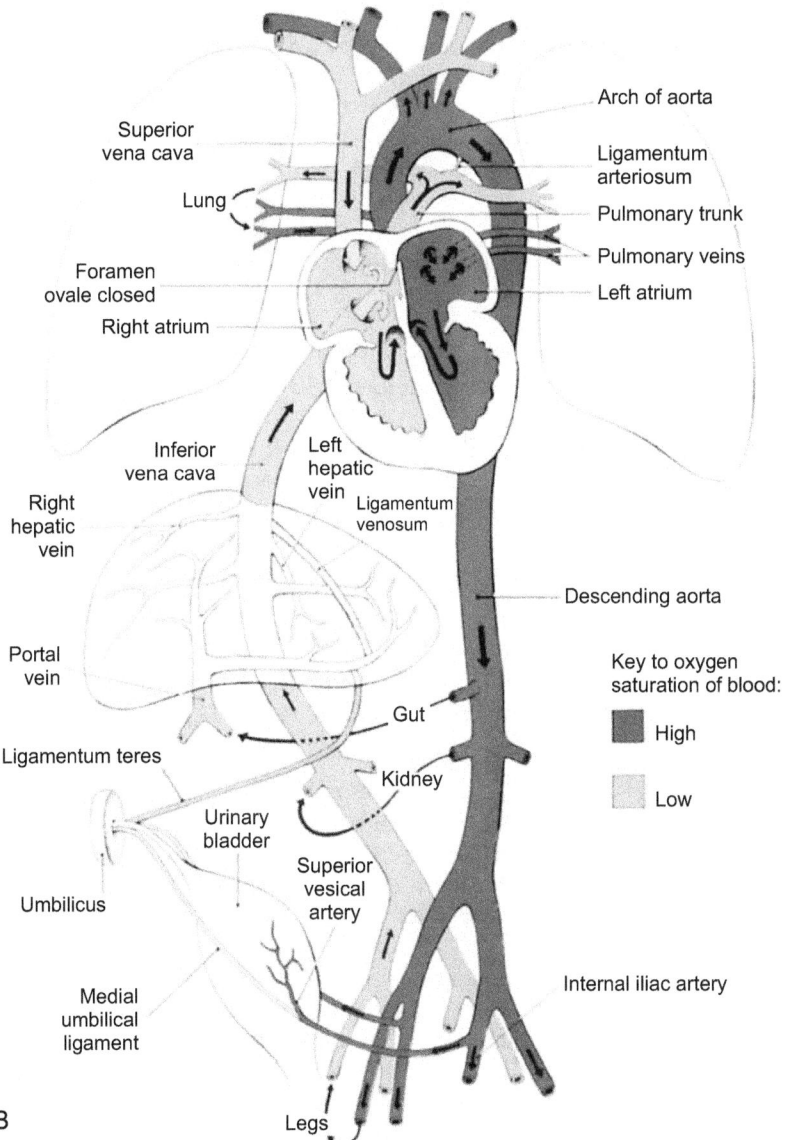

Figure 1-8, cont'd. B, Simplified representation of neonatal circulation. The adult derivatives of the fetal vessels and structures that become nonfunctional at birth are shown, and the arrows indicate the course of neonatal circulation. The organs are not drawn to scale. After birth, the three shunts that short-circuited the blood during fetal life cease to function, and the pulmonary and systemic circulations become separated. (From Moore KL, Persaud TVN: **The developing human: clinically oriented embryology,** ed 6, Philadelphia, 1998, WB Saunders.)

the wall separating the left and right atria. Before birth, the stream of blood flowing into the heart from the inferior vena cava is divided between the right and left atria by part of the atrial septum, the upper edge of the septum primum. There is more oxygen (less venous admixture) in the left atrium, because the flow of highly oxygenated blood from the inferior vena cava is diluted by only a small amount of deoxygenated blood from the fetal lungs. After birth, pressure in the left atrium rises because of increased left atrial blood flow from increased pulmonary venous return. Right atrial pressure falls because of decreased pulmonary vascular resistance. The atrial septum, which is constructed like a one-way valve (Figure 1-8, B), closes, preventing backflow of blood from left to right. In 10% of children with congenital heart disease who survive infancy, blood continues to flow via the foramen ovale across the atrial septum because of an **atrial septal defect** (ASD). This anomaly is described in Chapter 11.

During fetal life, the blood flow across the foramen ovale is right to left; postnatally, the flow is usually left to right. In those situations in which right atrial pressure exceeds left atrial pressure, as in severe pulmonic stenosis or pulmonary atresia, tricuspid atresia, or persistent pulmonary hypertension, blood continues to flow right to left in postnatal life across an atrial septal defect.

COMMUNICATIONS BETWEEN SYSTEMIC AND PULMONARY CIRCULATIONS

Communications between the systemic and pulmonary circulations, both within the heart and outside of it, are essential in prenatal life. After birth, such communications are called **shunts**. Shunts effectively short-circuit the flowing blood and prevent it from following its normal pathway. A shunt is described as left-to-right if the short circuit is from the arterial to the venous part of the circulation, or right-to-left if it is from the venous to the arterial part.

Shunts are further divided into those within the heart (intracardiac) and those outside it (extracardiac). Intracardiac shunts may result from defects in either the atrial or ventricular septum. In some cases, the defect is an isolated one; in others, it is part of a complex abnormality, such as a common atrioventricular canal. Extracardiac shunts can be caused by a patent ductus arteriosus, an abnormal opening in the septum between the aorta and the pulmonary artery, a pulmonary artery arising from the ascending aorta, a sinus of Valsalva fistula, an arteriovenous communication, or surgical intervention. Any of these abnormalities may cause murmurs and are discussed in later chapters.

HEART FAILURE

The term **heart failure** simply means failure of the heart to pump enough

BOX 1-1	Features of Heart Failure in Infants

Poor feeding and failure to thrive
Respiratory distress—mainly tachypnea
Rapid heart rate (160 to 180 beats/min)
Pulmonary rales or wheezing
Cardiomegaly and pulmonary edema on radiogram
Hepatomegaly (peripheral edema unusual)
Gallop sounds
Color—ashen pale or faintly cyanotic
Excessive perspiration
Diminished urine output

From Friedman WF, Silverman N: Congenital heart disease in infancy and childhood. In Braunwald E, Zipes DP, Libby P, editors: **Heart Disease,** 6th ed. Philadelphia, WB Saunders, 2001.

blood to meet the metabolic needs of the body. In children, heart failure is usually the result of volume overload caused by shunts, which themselves result from congenital malformations of the heart. Heart failure may be manifested by either a decrease in cardiac output or damming of blood in the vessels leading to the left or right sides of the heart (even though the cardiac output may be normal).

Because the left and right sides of the heart are two distinct pumps, one may fail independently of the other. In adults, failure of the left side of the heart occurs 30 times more often than failure of the right side of the heart, usually the result of occlusion of a coronary artery and myocardial infarct. In children with congenital heart disease, right-sided heart failure may occur without any left-sided failure.

When the left side of the heart fails, the mean pulmonary filling pressure rises and the volume of blood in the lungs increases. The result is congestion of the pulmonary vessels and pulmonary edema. In children, the most common sign of pulmonary edema is rapid breathing (tachypnea) rather than cough or crackles in the lungs, as in adults.

Failure of the right side of the heart leads to a shift of blood from the lungs into the systemic circulation, and decreased cardiac output stimulates the kidneys to retain fluid. The most common manifestation of right-sided heart failure in children is enlargement of the liver (hepatomegaly). Box 1-1 summarizes the features of heart failure in infants.

BIBLIOGRAPHY

Friedman WF, Silverman N: Congenital heart disease in infancy and childhood. In Braunwald E, Zipes DP, Libby P, editors: **Heart disease,** ed 6, Philadelphia, 2001, WB Saunders.

Gleick J: Computers attack heart disease. **New York Times,** August 5, 1986, p C1.

Guyton AC, Hall JE: **Textbook of medical physiology,** ed 10, Philadelphia, 2000, WB Saunders.

LeWinter MM, Osol G: Normal physiology of the cardiovascular system. In Fuster V, Alexander RW, O'Rourke RA, editors: **Hurst's the heart,** New York, 2001, McGraw Hill.

McKusick VA: **Cardiovascular sound in health and disease,** Baltimore, 1958, Williams & Wilkins.

McQueen DM, Peskin CS, Yellin EL: Fluid dynamics of the mitral valve: physiological aspects of a mathematical model, **Am J Physiol** 242:H1095-H1110, 1982.

Suga H: Cardiac function. In Moller JH, Hoffman JI, editors: **Pediatric cardiovascular medicine,** Philadelphia, 2000, Churchill Livingston.

Robinson TF, Factor SM, Sonnenblick EH: The heart as a suction pump, **Sci Am** 254:84-91, 1986.

Chapter 2

Sound, Hearing, and the Stethoscope

NATURE OF SOUND

Sounds are made up of audible vibrations created by alternating regions of compression and rarefaction of air. A tracing of a sound wave may be made by mounting a pen on one prong of a vibrating tuning fork and then running a piece of paper under the pen. The pen inscribes an S-shaped curve called a **sine wave.** The peaks and valleys in the wave correspond to the alternating regions of compression and rarefaction that make up the sound wave (Figure 2-1).

Sound has three principal characteristics: frequency, intensity, and duration (Figure 2-2). **Frequency** is a measure of the number of vibrations per unit time, in cycles per second, or hertz (Hz). A large number of vibrations, as in a high-frequency murmur, yield a sound that is subjectively interpreted as being high-pitched. Alternatively, a low-frequency murmur gives a sound that is perceived as low-pitched.

Intensity is governed by four factors: (1) the amplitude of the vibrations, (2) the source producing the energy, (3) the distance the vibrations must travel, and (4) the medium through which they travel. These factors determine whether a sound, such as a heart murmur, is perceived as loud or faint.

Duration of the vibrations determines whether the ear interprets them as short or long, for example, a short murmur or a long one.

A fourth characteristic, **quality** (also known as **timbre**), is a result of the component frequencies that make up any particular sound. The quality of the sound is what makes a note played on the violin perceptibly different from the same note played on a piano (Figure 2-3). For heart murmurs, quality provides a distinction between a harsh murmur and a musical one.

Musical notes and heart sounds are made up of several frequency components. In a musical note, each of these components, which are simple multiples of one another, is called a **harmonic.** In most heart sounds, the relationship of the components is more complex, although some murmurs are quite analogous to musical notes. The pitch of a sound is determined by

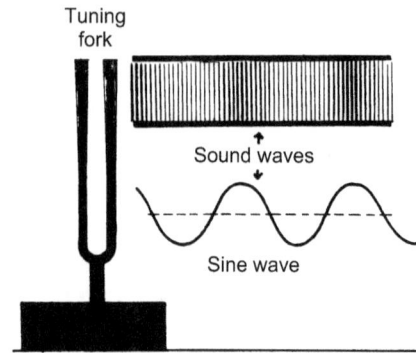

FIGURE 2-1. The vibrating tuning fork produces the sound wave **(top),** which consists of alternating areas of compressed and rarefied air. The changing pressure in these areas corresponds to the sine wave below. (From Rushmer RF: **Cardiac diagnosis: a physiologic approach,** Philadelphia, 1955, WB Saunders.)

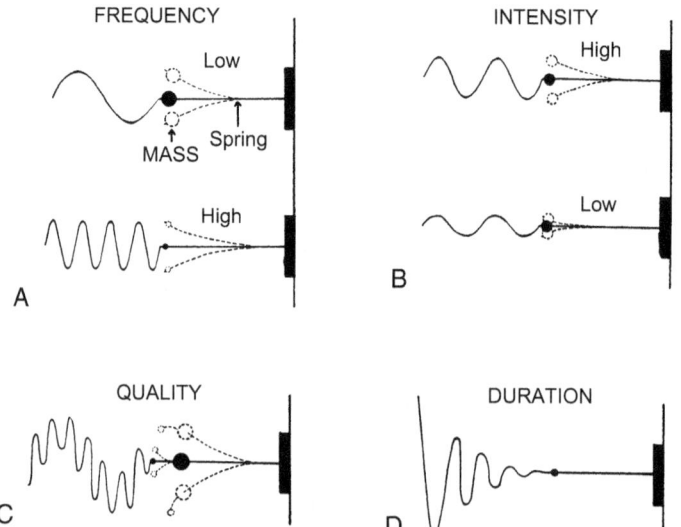

FIGURE 2-2. A, The frequency of vibration is determined by the relationship between mass and elasticity of the vibrating body. As shown in the example here, the larger mass **(upper drawing)** vibrates at a lower frequency. **B,** The amplitude of the vibration and the corresponding intensity of the sound depend on the amount of displacement of the vibrating body; a high-intensity sound is produced by a large displacement **(upper drawing). C,** The quality, or timbre, of the sound is a result of the relative intensity of the component frequencies that make up the vibration. Shown here is a high-frequency sine wave (overtone) superimposed on a low-frequency sine wave (the fundamental). **D,** The duration of a vibration after the source of energy is cut off is dependent on the level of the energy and the rate at which it is dissipated. Note that each peak in the sine wave, going from left to right, is lower than the one before, indicating that the sound is diminishing progressively in amplitude. (From Rushmer RF: **Cardiac diagnosis: a physiologic approach,** Philadelphia, 1955, WB Saunders.)

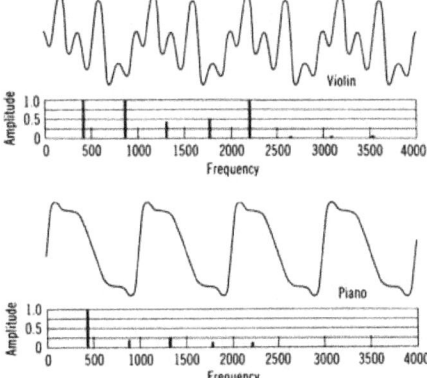

FIGURE 2-3. Wave form and sound spectrum for two stringed instruments, the violin and the piano. The fundamental frequency for both is 440 Hz (concert A). Four cycles of each wave are shown. The sound spectrum beneath each wave demonstrates the harmonic components of the wave. Note the presence of loud higher harmonics, especially the fifth, in the violin spectrum. (From Halliday D, Resnick R: **Physics,** New York, 1966, Wiley.)

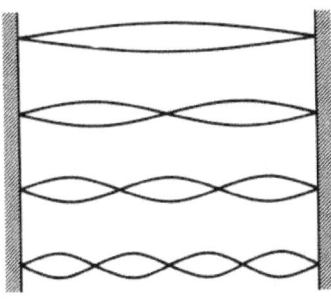

FIGURE 2-4. A vibrating string, fixed at both ends, showing the first four modes of vibration. The uppermost mode produces the fundamental tone; the lower three modes generate the overtones. (From Halliday D, Resnick R: **Physics,** New York, 1966, Wiley.)

the component of lowest frequency, called the **fundamental.** The quality of a sound is determined by the high-frequency components, called **overtones** in a musical sound (Figure 2-4). In music, frequency or pitch is often expressed in terms of octaves above or below a given pitch, such as middle C. In the case of heart sounds, the number of cycles per second (Hz) is the preferred unit of measure.

HEARING

Most heart sounds fall into a frequency range to which the ear is relatively insensitive. Some basic physiology of hearing may clarify this point.

The eardrum is mechanically attached to the cochlear apparatus by three tiny bones of the middle ear (the malleus, incus, and stapes), called the **ossicles** (Figure 2-5). The cochlea is essentially a selective sound frequency transducer, and a remarkably sensitive one. The eardrum needs to move only a distance equal to one tenth the diameter of a hydrogen molecule for sound to be heard.

The average young, healthy ear can detect sound vibrations with frequencies between approximately 16 and 16,000 Hz, although sensitivity

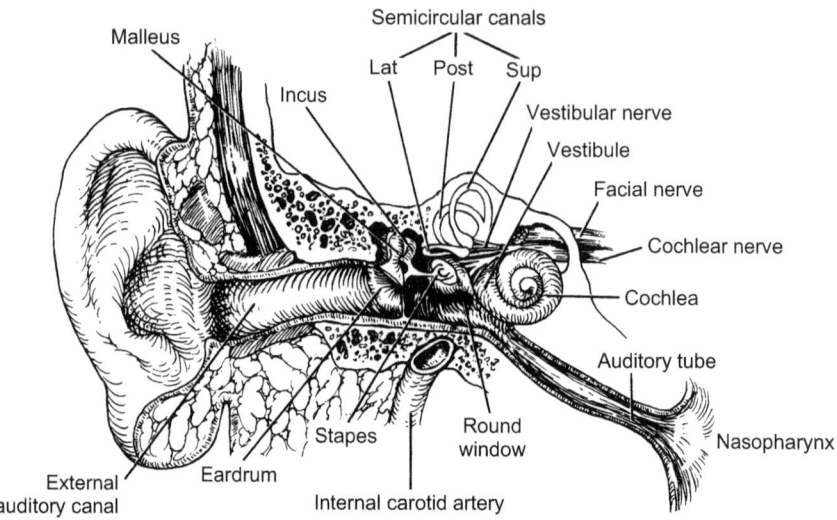

FIGURE 2-5. The human ear. Sound waves pass through the external auditory canal inward to the tympanic membrane, or eardrum. The middle ear is an air-filled cavity in the temporal bone that opens to the outside via the auditory tube and nasopharynx; the tube is usually closed. The three ossicles—the malleus, incus, and stapes—are located in the middle ear. The manubrium, or handle, of the malleus is attached to the back of the tympanic membrane; its head is attached to the wall of the middle ear, and its short process is attached to the incus, which in turn is joined to the head of the stapes (named for its resemblance to a stirrup). The faceplate of the stapes lies against the oval window; sound waves are transmitted from here into the cochlea. To make the relationships clear, the cochlea has been turned slightly and the middle ear muscles have been omitted. **Lat,** Lateral; **post,** posterior; **sup,** superior. (From Brödel M: **Three unpublished drawings of the anatomy of the human ear.** Philadelphia, 1946, WB Saunders.)

varies greatly through this range. Maximum sensitivity is in the region of 1000 to 2000 Hz. Below 1000 Hz sensitivity falls off dramatically. For example, to be audible, a tone with a frequency of 100 Hz must have a sound pressure 100 times greater than a tone at 1000 Hz. Because most normal heart sounds are below 500 Hz, the ear is relatively insensitive to them, and they are not heard as well as other types of sound (Figure 2-6).

The **Fletcher-Munson phenomenon** further complicates the frequency response characteristics of the ear. At a high level of absolute intensity, sounds are more likely to be perceived by the ear as equally loud, regardless of frequency composition. At a low level of absolute intensity, sounds seem to the ear to be high-pitched. Although the Fletcher-Munson phenomenon is not a factor when a stethoscope is being used, it does affect the perception of recorded heart sounds played through a speaker. These sounds seem unnaturally low-pitched and booming to the ear when compared with heart sounds heard through a stethoscope. Therefore, the heart sounds CD accompanying this book should be listened to through a stethoscope, with the bell held 2 to 3 inches from the speaker of the CD player.

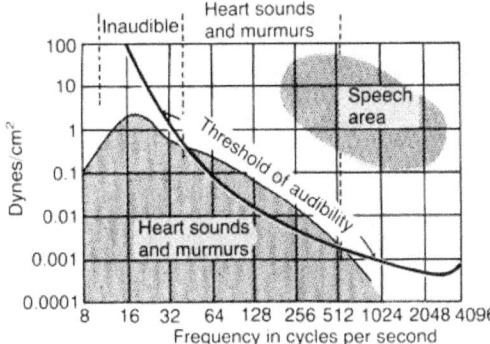

FIGURE 2-6. Amplitude of different frequency vibrations in heart sounds and heart murmurs in relation to the threshold of audibility, showing that the range of sounds that can be heard is between about 40 and 500 cycles per second. (From Guyton AC, Hall JE: **Textbook of medical physiology,** ed 10, Philadelphia, 2000, WB Saunders.)

Because other sensory stimuli occurring during auscultation may dull auditory perception, reducing interference from such stimuli to a minimum is important. A good clinician listening for a faint sound through the stethoscope seeks as quiet a room as possible.

THE STETHOSCOPE

Clinicians have listened to the sounds within the chest since antiquity. Until the nineteenth century, these sounds were detected by listening with the ear placed directly against the chest wall (Figure 2-7), despite the obvious drawbacks of a patient's desire for modesty or aversion to contact. In 1816, faced with examining the chest of an obese woman, a French physician, René Théophile Laënnec, devised an alternative. He rolled a sheaf of paper into a cylinder, placed one end on the patient's chest, and put his ear to the other end (Figure 2-8). Laënnec named his invention the stethoscope, from the Greek **stethos** (breast) and **skopein** (to view). Subsequently, he employed a wooden cylinder, and in 1819 he published a treatise on what he had learned with his instrument.

The modern stethoscope is usually a combination of tubing, a binaural headset, eartips, and two types of chest pieces (Figure 2-9). For best results, these elements must all function properly, and the stethoscope must fit the ears well.

The open **bell,** or Ford chest piece, is similar to the old-fashioned trumpet-type hearing aid. It conducts sound with practically no distortion, but it makes all sounds loud. Because low-frequency sounds are hard to hear, the bell is well suited for them. The bell is not recommended for listening to high-frequency sounds.

The closed **diaphragm,** or Bowles chest piece, has a larger diameter than the bell. Because it acts to attenuate low-frequency sounds and pass high-frequency sounds, it is best suited for hearing high-pitched sounds.

It is important to note that the bell chest piece functions as a diaphragm

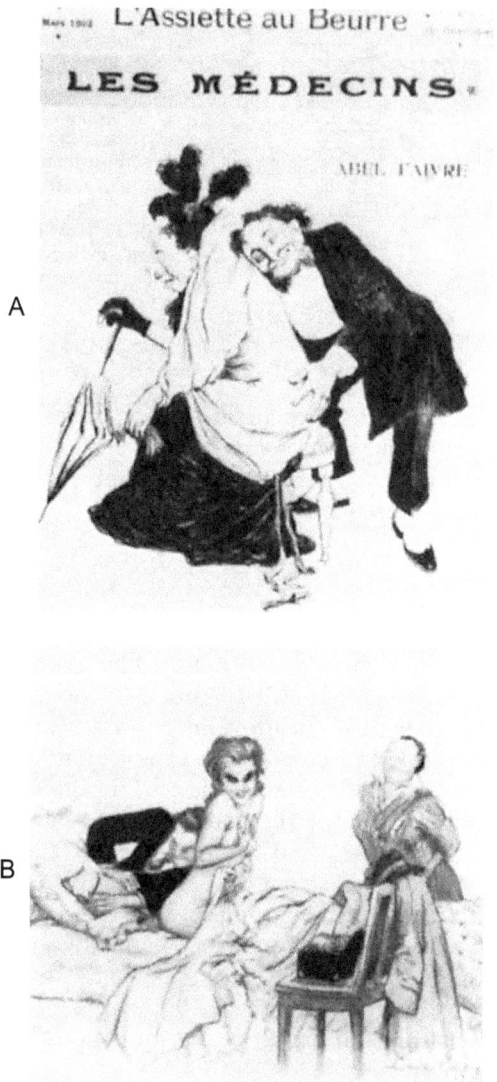

FIGURE 2-7. **A** and **B,** Direct auscultation of the chest, portrayed in two French caricatures. (From McKusick VA: **Cardiovascular sound in health and disease,** Baltimore, 1958, Williams & Wilkins.)

chest piece when applied too tightly to the skin. The skin acts as the diaphragm, and low-frequency sounds are more difficult to discern.

The binaurals should be light and comfortable. The eartubes must be inclined anteriorly to conform to the direction of the normal ear canals. The importance of a snug yet gentle fit at the ears cannot be overemphasized. Even

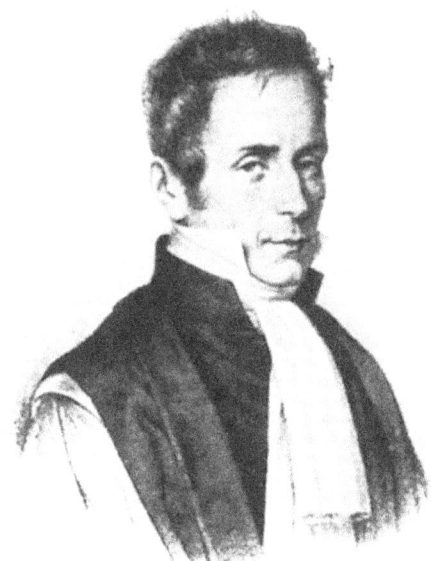

FIGURE 2-8. René Théophile Laënnec (1781-1826) was the French physician who invented the stethoscope and gave the first accurate descriptions of normal and abnormal breath sounds, correlating them with pathologic autopsy findings. (From Garrison FH: **An introduction to the history of medicine,** ed 4, Philadelphia, 1929, WB Saunders.)

A

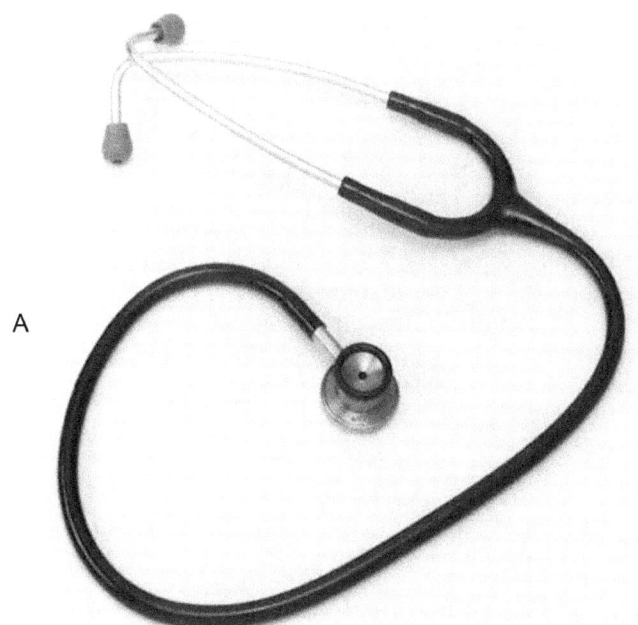

FIGURE 2-9. A, An infant stethoscope.

Continued

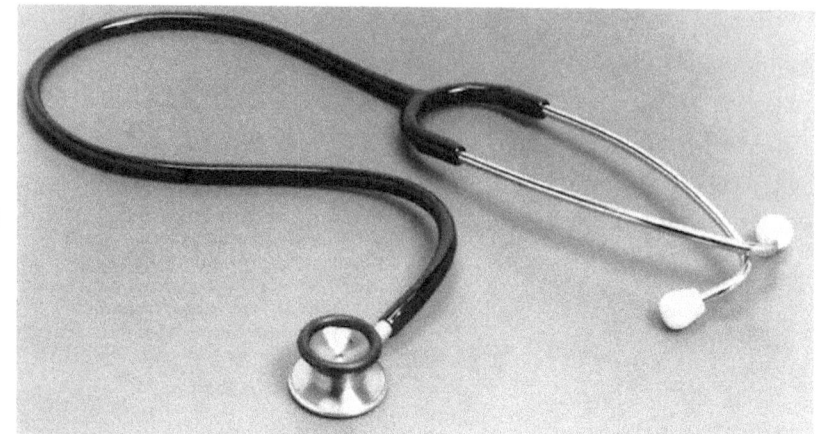

B

FIGURE 2-9, cont'd. B, A pediatric stethoscope. (Courtesy 3M Company.)

the best chest piece is completely unsatisfactory when joined to an uncomfortable headset and poorly fitting eartips.

The stethoscope should be well maintained and cared for. Broken diaphragms should not be replaced by or improvised from x-ray film, for example, which is a poor diaphragm substitute. A Bowles chest piece with either a makeshift or absent diaphragm is a very poor instrument. Moreover, replacing the original flexible tubing with hospital tubing intended for other purposes is not advisable.

In pediatrics, two specialized stethoscopes are used. A regular pediatric stethoscope has a smaller chest piece than the adult model, and a stethoscope with an even smaller chest piece is used for examining premature infants. The tubing is also longer so that it can reach inside an incubator.

In a very thin child, especially if the stethoscope chest piece is relatively large, complete apposition of the diaphragm to the chest wall may be difficult to achieve. The result of incomplete apposition is a harsh noise, generated by intermittent contact of skin with the diaphragm of the stethoscope, especially at the cardiac apex. The harsh noise can sound like a pericardial friction rub.

BIBLIOGRAPHY

Guyton AC, Hall JE: **Textbook of medical physiology,** ed 10, Philadelphia, 2000, WB Saunders.

Kindig JR, Beeson TP, Campbell RW et al: Acoustical performance of the stethoscope: a comparative analysis, **Am Heart J** 104:269-275, 1982.

Littmann D: Stethoscopes and auscultation, **Am J Nurs** 72:1238-1241, 1972.

McKusick VA: **Cardiovascular sound in health and disease,** Baltimore, 1958, Williams & Wilkins.

Moller JH: Clinical history and physical examination. In Moller JH, Hoffman JI, editors: **Pediatric cardiovascular medicine,** Philadelphia, 2000, Churchill Livingston.

Rappaport MB, Sprague HB: The effects of tubing bore on stethoscope efficiency, **Am Heart J** 42:605, 1951.

Reiser SJ: The medical influence of the stethoscope, **Sci Am** 240:148-156, 1979.

Chapter 3

History and Physical Examination of the Child With Heart Disease

A careful history and physical examination form the basis for all diagnosis of heart disease by health care personnel. Indeed, the assessment data obtained may be the only readily available information, particularly for a new patient or a child seen without a parent—in school, for example. The results of a careful history and physical examination often suggest further tests that should be performed.

HISTORY

Careful interviewing of the child and/or caregiver is essential in obtaining a complete history. In addition to identifying data (child's age, date of birth, sex, and so on), information should be gathered about the chief complaint, the prenatal history, birth and postnatal history, and family history.

Chief Complaint

The chief complaint is a concise description of the reason for the referral for a cardiac examination, and the most important question to be answered is whether the child has symptoms of heart disease. Information gathered should include how sick the child is and which, if any, of the complaints may result from previous discovery of a cardiac problem. The appearance of a child who is sick "because the doctor said so," or whose exercise limitation results from parental restriction because the child is "too active," is entirely different from that of the child who "does not gain weight or grow like others," who "turns blue," who "breathes heavily," or who "cannot keep up." The former child may have only a benign murmur, whereas the latter most probably has serious heart disease.

In newborns or small infants, the chief complaint of a heart murmur, especially if associated with cyanosis or heart failure, may be the result of complex congenital heart disease (see Chapter 15). The range of possible

27

symptoms is quite small.

In an older infant or child, the cause of a murmur is more likely to be a single lesion, or the murmur may be innocent and not reflect the presence of any heart disease. In older children, acquired lesions (resulting from rheumatic fever, for example, or from subacute bacterial endocarditis often secondary to congenital heart disease) are more common.

Prenatal History

A number of prenatal conditions may predispose the infant or child to cardiac disease.

Infection

Maternal infection may result in several types of cardiac problems in newborns. Rubella (German measles) during the first 3 months of pregnancy often results in multiple fetal abnormalities, among them cardiac defects. Similarly, maternal infection in early pregnancy with cytomegalovirus, herpesvirus, or coxsackievirus B may cause congenital heart defects. Infections with these viruses later in pregnancy may cause myocarditis. Smallpox vaccination during pregnancy may also cause congenital malformations.

Fetal Alcohol Syndrome

High levels of alcohol ingested by the mother during pregnancy damage the embryo and interfere with fetal development. The greater the alcohol intake, the more severe the damage: 32% of infants born to heavy drinkers have congenital abnormalities, compared with 14% born to moderate drinkers and 9% to abstainers. Fetal alcohol syndrome appears in 1 or 2 infants per 1000 live births. The characteristics of fetal alcohol syndrome include (1) prenatal onset of growth deficiency; (2) facial abnormalities; (3) cardiac defects, primarily septal defects; (4) minor joint and limb abnormalities; and (5) delayed mental development and mental retardation.

Drugs

Various medications may cause birth defects. Drugs used to control epileptic seizures (e.g., hydantoin or trimethadione), if taken by a pregnant woman, may cause congenital heart disease. Retinoic acid (Accutane), used in the treatment of severe cystic acne, has produced many serious birth defects. Smoking can cause low birth weight. A careful history of maternal exposure during the first 2 to 8 weeks after conception is important.

Illness

Maternal illness is associated with several cardiac defects. Infants of diabetic mothers may have abnormalities of the heart, and maternal lupus erythematosus can produce congenital heart block in infants (see Chapter 6). The risk of cardiac defects also increases (to 10% or 15%) if the mother has congenital heart disease.

Certain genetic diseases (Marfan, Holt-Oram, and Williams syndrome) are associated with heart deformities. These conditions are inherited as autosomal dominant traits. Children with Alagille syndrome, caused by a defect in chromosome 20p11-12, have peripheral pulmonary arterial stenoses, biliary dysfunction, and facial abnormalities. In addition, there is a high prevalence of congenital heart disease in children with chromosomal abnormalities, such as Down syndrome (trisomy 21), trisomy 13 and 18, and Turner syndrome. Many cavotruncal abnormalities are associated with the cardiovelofacial syndrome (caused by a deletion on chromosome 22).

Weight and Prematurity

Birth weight may suggest the cause of a cardiac abnormality. Low birth weight (being small for gestational age) may be the result of a maternal infection, which in turn may be associated with cardiac abnormalities. Prematurity is associated with patent ductus arteriosus. High birth weight (being large for gestational age) often occurs in infants of diabetic mothers and is also associated with transposition of the great arteries. Infants with transposition are cyanotic at birth.

Birth and Past Health History

Birth

Information about the delivery (for example, vaginal or cesarean) should be obtained. The examiner should ascertain whether the infant was cyanotic at birth, whether any resuscitative measures were used, and whether oxygen was administered. If the baby's discharge from the hospital was delayed, congenital heart disease might have been present.

Development

Failure to gain weight, developmental problems, and feeding problems may be associated with congestive heart failure and severe cyanosis. Weight gain is affected more than height. In early congestive heart failure, babies feed poorly because of fatigue and shortness of breath. These infants often gain weight adequately with good care but take longer to feed than a normal infant, sometimes as long as 40 minutes per feeding.

Cyanosis, Hypoxic Spells, and Squatting

Cyanosis, hypoxic spells, and squatting are signs of congenital heart disease. If the parents have noted **cyanosis,** it is important to determine whether it began in the hospital nursery or after the child came home and to establish its severity. (Is it permanent or episodic? What parts of the body become cyanotic? Does the cyanosis become worse after feeding?) It is important to be aware that parents may not recognize cyanosis if it is mild and the child is their first or has dark skin.

Hypoxic spells are characterized by a period of uncontrollable crying, followed by paroxysms of shortness of breath, cyanosis, unconsciousness, or seizures. Hypoxic spells, which are potentially fatal and constitute a medical emergency, are commonly associated with tetralogy of Fallot (see Chapter 15). The parents should be asked when the spells occur (when the infant feeds or on awakening in the morning), how long the spells last, and how often they occur. It is important to establish whether the infant breathes quickly and deeply during the spells, or if the breath is held. Breath-holding spells, although frightening, are distinct from hypoxic spells and are not in themselves dangerous, nor are they symptomatic of heart disease.

Squatting is often a sign of cyanotic heart disease, especially tetralogy of Fallot. Ask the parents if the child squats when tired.

Respiratory Symptoms

Rapid breathing **(tachypnea)** and shortness of breath **(dyspnea)** are the main signs of congestive heart failure in children. Puffy eyelids, also a sign of congestive heart failure, may or may not be present. Tachypnea is worse during feeding, and feeding and weight gain are poor. Wheezing and persistent night cough may also be signs of early congestive heart failure but are more likely caused by allergies. Ankle edema, a sign of congestive heart failure in adults, is rarely seen in children.

Lower respiratory infections, especially bronchitis or pneumonia, are frequent in congenital heart disease, particularly in children with large left-to-right shunts. Upper respiratory infections have no relationship to congenital heart disease.

Diminished **exercise tolerance** is often a sign of congenital heart disease. The parents should be asked whether the child keeps up with others, how many blocks the child can walk or run, and how many flights of stairs the child can climb without excessive fatigue.

Heart Murmur

When a heart murmur is the chief complaint, it is helpful to have the following information about the circumstances of its discovery:

1. Was the murmur present at birth? If not, how long after birth was it discovered? A heart murmur heard within a few hours of birth may be caused by aortic or pulmonic valve stenosis. A small left-to-right shunt through a ventricular septal defect or patent ductus arteriosus may not produce an audible murmur for a few days or weeks.
2. Was the murmur discovered by a clinician who had been caring for the child for some time or by a new caregiver who was seeing the child for the first time? A heart murmur first noted during routine examination of a healthy-looking child is likely to be innocent, especially if noted by the child's regular caregiver. In a child older than 5 years, the murmur

could be the result of rheumatic fever.
3. Did the child have a febrile illness immediately preceding the appearance of the murmur? Heart murmurs are often discovered during a febrile illness.
4. Did the child have episodes of sore throat at any time before the murmur was detected? If so, the murmur may be the result of rheumatic heart disease.

Precise information regarding these four points is vital and may be the only clue allowing differentiation between congenital heart disease, present from birth, and acquired heart disease, such as rheumatic heart disease, which often follows a febrile illness and, particularly, a sore throat.

Chest Pain
Chest pain is uncommon in children and is not usually related to heart disease. Some heart conditions do cause chest pain in children. **Aortic stenosis** produces pain during activity. The pain associated with **mitral valve prolapse** (see Chapters 9 and 11) does not accompany activity. Rarely, chest pain is caused by **severe pulmonic valve stenosis, pericarditis,** and **Kawasaki disease** (an acute inflammatory illness usually found in infants or small children and characterized by high fever and inflammation of the mouth and conjunctiva). Two percent of children with Kawasaki disease die because of sudden inflammation of the blood vessels of the heart, which causes myocardial infarction.

To determine the source of chest pain in children, the following information should be obtained. The person taking the history should determine whether the child has the pain only when active or whether pain also occurs when the child is at rest. Information about the duration of the pain (minutes, seconds, hours), the character of the pain (stabbing, squeezing), and its distribution (Does it radiate to other parts of the body, such as the neck, shoulder, or left arm?) may also be helpful in determining its cause. Ascertaining whether the pain is associated with fainting or palpitations and whether deep breathing reduces or increases it is important. Pain of cardiac origin, with the exception of pericarditis, is not influenced by deep breathing. Mindful of heredity, the examiner should also ask whether there has been a recent cardiac death in the family that was preceded by complaints of chest pain.

Medications
Medications can produce cardiac symptoms in the absence of heart disease. Tachycardia and palpitations can be caused by antiasthmatic drugs, such as aminophylline, or by cold medications.

Rheumatic Fever
Until recently, rheumatic fever was all but eradicated in the United States. At

one time, however, entire hospitals were devoted to the care of patients with rheumatic fever and rheumatic heart disease. With the discovery of the role **Streptococcus** type A plays in the development of rheumatic fever, and the treatment of streptococcal sore throat with antibiotics, rheumatic fever can be prevented in most cases.

Since 1988, rheumatic fever has experienced a resurgence. Some hospitals that had only a handful of patients a year are now reporting a significantly increased incidence. Although rheumatic fever is not an epidemic yet, it is making a comeback, and the reasons are unknown.

This reappearance of what was once a major debilitating childhood illness is cause for concern. Almost half of all children with rheumatic fever suffer permanent, sometimes fatal, heart damage.

In a child with **joint symptoms,** therefore, the possibility and diagnosis of rheumatic fever must be recognized. Joint symptoms should be investigated by asking about the number of joints affected, the duration of the symptoms, and whether the pain migrates from joint to joint or is stationary. The joint pain in acute rheumatic fever is usually very severe. If the child complaining of joint pain can walk, rheumatic fever can probably be ruled out. Because aspirin and other salicylates can suppress or eliminate the joint pain of rheumatic fever, whether the child received aspirin and, if so, how much and how often is an important part of the history. The examiner should determine whether the joints are swollen, red, hot, or tender and whether the child has had abdominal or chest pain (suggestive of pericarditis) or nosebleeds. All are associated with rheumatic fever.

Whether the child had a recent sore throat and whether a throat culture was taken are important questions to ask. Although a diagnosis of rheumatic fever requires a preceding infection with **Streptococcus** type A, a third of patients with acute rheumatic fever cannot recall having a sore throat. Two to four weeks after infection, the cardinal signs of rheumatic fever (the **major criteria of Jones**) plus a number of minor criteria appear (Box 3-1). Evidence of a preceding streptococcal infection and either one major and two minor criteria or two major criteria must be present to establish a diagnosis of rheumatic fever.

Neurologic Symptoms

Neurologic symptoms may be a clue to underlying cardiac disease. If the child has experienced episodes of "stroke," neurologic symptoms may be caused by endocarditis or severe cyanotic heart disease. Headaches, personality changes, or somnolence, particularly in an older child with a right-to-left shunt, may indicate a brain abscess. In adolescents with coarctation of the aorta (see Chapter 11) or polycythemia, headaches are a common complaint. Weakness and poor coordination might suggest myocardiopathy associated with Friedreich's ataxia or muscular dystrophy. Choreiform movement (spasmodic twitching) may result from rheumatic fever.

BOX 3-1	Guidelines for the Diagnosis of Initial Attack of Rheumatic Fever (Jones Criteria, 1992 Update)*

Major Manifestations
Carditis
Polyarthritis
Chorea
Erythema marginatum
Subcutaneous nodules

Minor Manifestations
Clinical findings
   Previous rheumatic fever or rheumatic heart disease
   Arthralgia
   Fever
Laboratory findings
   Acute phase reactants
      Erythrocyte sedimentation rate
      C-reactive protein, leukocytosis
   Prolonged PR interval

Supporting Evidence of Streptococcal Infection
Increased titer of streptococcal antibodies
   ASO (antistreptolysin O)
   Other antibodies
Positive throat culture for group A **Streptococcus**
Recent scarlet fever

From Guidelines for the diagnosis of rheumatic fever, **JAMA** 268:2070, 1992. Copyright 1992, American Medical Association.
*The presence of two major criteria or of one major and two minor criteria indicates a high probability of the presence of rheumatic fever. Evidence of a preceding streptococcal infection greatly strengthens the possibility of acute rheumatic fever; its absence should make the diagnosis doubtful (except in Sydenham's chorea or long-standing carditis).

Syncope (fainting) can be caused by abnormal cardiac rhythms (particularly abnormal ventricular rhythms), by mitral valve prolapse, and by severe aortic stenosis (during activity only). However, most syncope in children is unrelated to heart disease. The following must be ruled out:

Long QT Syndrome. This condition is inherited and is characterized by syncope, seizures, and sudden death. Most affected children exhibit a prolongation of the QT interval on the electrocardiogram, along with bizarre or notched T waves and prominent U waves or T-wave alternans. Patients develop life-threatening ventricular tachycardia (called torsades de pointes) or ventricular fibrillation. Common presenting symptoms are listed in Table 3-1.

Children often present to a cardiac clinic with chest pain or a combination of dizziness and syncope. If the child has no history of chest pain and no arrhythmia, the complaint of pain may be a cry for more attention rather than a symptom of disease. Likewise, the complaints of dizziness and syncope are often unrelated to any cardiac pathologic condition. The child may have stood up too quickly in school and experienced vasovagal

TABLE 3–1. Presentation of Children with Long QT Syndrome

Presentation	Percentage
Cardiac arrest	9
Syncope	26
Seizures	10
Presyncope or palpitations	6
Family history	39
Asymptomatic	39

Modified from Vetter V: Arrhythmias. In Moller JH, Hoffman JI, editors: **Pediatric cardiovascular medicine,** Philadelphia, 2000, Churchill Livingston.

syncope, or have fainted on a warm day after prolonged standing, whereupon the school nurse immediately called the mother. Some clinicians may use a tilt table to try to reproduce the syncope.

Family History

The family history can be very helpful in evaluating a child with cardiac disease. Table 3-2 lists hereditary syndromes in which congenital heart disease is a common finding. The presence of congenital heart disease in a family member increases the likelihood that the child will be affected. With no family history, congenital heart disease occurs in 8 of 1000 live births, or at a rate of about 1%. Table 3-3 lists the relative frequency of specific cardiac malformations at birth.

Rheumatic fever is often seen in more than one family member. Although susceptibility to rheumatic fever appears to have a genetic component, a streptococcal infection must be present for the disease to occur.

PHYSICAL EXAMINATION

When examining a child, especially a small child or infant, the clinician must take care not to provoke a fit of crying. It is impossible to listen to the heart of a screaming child. A small child can be examined in the mother's lap, an infant in the mother's arms. An older child may be less apprehensive if first examined sitting rather than lying down. Above all, the examiner must remain calm, or the child will feel threatened and become uncooperative. Engaging the child in the examination as much as possible may help to reduce the child's concern, as may talking about school or other interests.

The traditional head-to-toe approach to physical examination is often not feasible with children. Instead, the clinician starts first with those parts of the examination that do not require the child's cooperation and then proceeds to the more difficult tasks. For example, beginning with an ear examination, which may be painful, can provoke crying or hysterics. It is best to start by

Text continued on p. 39

TABLE 3–2. Syndromes with Associated Cardiovascular Involvement

Syndrome	Major Cardiovascular Manifestations/(Genetic Locus)	Major Noncardiac Abnormalities
Heritable and Possibly Heritable/(Genetic Locus)		
Ellis-van Creveld	Single atrium or atrial septal defect	Chondrodystrophic dwarfism, nail dysplasia, polydactyly
TAR (thrombocytopenia–absent radius)	Atrial septal defect, tetralogy of Fallot	Radial aplasia or hypoplasia, thrombocytopenia
Holt-Oram	Atrial septal defect (other defects common) (12q21–q3)	Skeletal upper limb defect, hypoplasia of clavicles
Kartagener	Dextrocardia	Situs inversus, sinusitis, bronchiectasis
Laurence-Moon-Biedl-Bardet	Variable defects	Retinal pigmentation, obesity, polydactyly
Noonan	Pulmonic valve dysplasia, cardiomyopathy (usually hypertrophic) (12Q24)	Webbed neck, pectus excavatum, cryptorchidism
Tuberous sclerosis	Rhabdomyoma, cardiomyopathy (type 1–9q, type 2–16p)	Phakomatosis, bone lesions, hamartomatous skin lesions
Multiple lentigines (LEOPARD)	Pulmonic stenosis	Basal cell nevi, broad facies, rib anomalies, deafness
Rubinstein-Taybi	Patent ductus arteriosus (others) (16p13.3)	Broad thumbs and toes, hypoplastic maxilla, slanted palpebral fissures
Familial deafness	Arrhythmias, sudden death	Sensorineural deafness
Weber-Osler-Rendu	Arteriovenous fistulas (lung, liver, mucous membranes) (9q33–4)	Multiple telangiectasias
Apert	Ventricular septal defect (10q26)	Craniosynostosis, midfacial hypoplasia, syndactyly
Crouzon	Patent ductus arteriosus, aortic coarctation (10q26, 4p16.3)	Ptosis with shallow orbits, craniosynostosis, maxillary hypoplasia
Hypertrophic cardiomyopathy	Asymmetric septal hypertrophy (locus heterogeneity, 14q11.2–12, 1q32, 15.q22, 11p11.2, and others)	Family history of sudden death
Incontinentia pigmenti	Patent ductus arteriosus	Irregular pigmented skin lesions, patchy alopecia, hypodontia
Alagille (arteriohepatic dysplasia)	Peripheral pulmonic stenosis, pulmonic stenosis (20p12)	Biliary hypoplasia, vertebral anomalies, prominent forehead, deep-set eyes
Catch-22 (DiGeorge)	Interrupted aortic arch, tetralogy of Fallot, truncus arteriosus (22q11)	Thymic hypoplasia or aplasia, parathyroid aplasia or hypoplasia, abnormal facies
Shprintzen (velocardiofacial)	Ventricular septal defect, tetralogy of Fallot, right aortic arch (22q11.2)	Cleft palate, prominent nose, slender hands, learning disability

Continued

TABLE 3-2—cont'd

Syndrome	Major Cardiovascular Manifestations	Major Noncardiac Abnormalities
Williams	Supravalvular aortic stenosis, peripheral pulmonic stenosis (7q11.23)	Mental deficiency, elfin facies, loquacious personality, hoarse voice
Long Q-T (Jervell and Lange-Nielsen, Romano-Ward)	Long QT interval, ventricular arrhythmias (11p15.5, 7q35, 3p21, 21q22)	Family history of sudden death, congenital deafness (not in Romano-Ward)
Friedreich's ataxia	Cardiomyopathy and conduction defects (9q)	Ataxia, speech defect, degeneration of spinal cord dorsal columns
Muscular dystrophy	Cardiomyopathy	Pseudohypertrophy of calf muscles, weakness of trunk and proximal limb muscles
Cystic fibrosis	Cor pulmonale (7q)	Pancreatic insufficiency, malabsorption, chronic lung disease
Sickle cell anemia	Cardiomyopathy, mitral regurgitation (11p)	Hemoglobin SS
Conradi-Hünermann	Ventricular septal defect, patent ductus arteriosus	Asymmetrical limb shortness, early punctate mineralization, large skin pores
Cockayne	Accelerated atherosclerosis	Cachectic dwarfism, retinal pigment abnormalities, photosensitivity dermatitis
Progeria	Accelerated atherosclerosis	Premature aging, alopecia, atrophy of subcutaneous fat, skeletal hypoplasia
Connective Tissue Disorders		
Cutis laxa	Peripheral pulmonic stenosis	Generalized disruption of elastic fibers, diminished skin resilience, hernias
Ehlers-Danlos	Arterial dilatation and rupture, mitral regurgitation (2q31)	Hyperextensible joints, hyperelastic and friable
Marfan	Aortic dilatation, aortic and mitral incompetence (15q21.1)	Gracile habitus, arachnodactyly with hyperextensibility, lens subluxation
Osteogenesis imperfecta	Aortic incompetence (7, 17)	Fragile bones, blue sclerae
Pseudoxanthoma elasticum	Peripheral and coronary arterial disease	Degeneration of elastic fibers in skin, retinal angioid streaks

Inborn Errors of Metabolism

Condition	Cardiac findings	Features
Pompe disease	Glycogen storage disease of heart	Acid maltase deficiency, muscle weakness
Homocystinuria	Aortic and pulmonary artery dilatation, intravascular thrombosis	Cystathionine b-synthase deficiency, lens subluxation, osteoporosis
Mucopolysaccharidoses: Hurler; Hunter	Multivalvular and coronary and great artery disease; cardiomyopathy	Hurler: Deficiency of α-L-iduronidase, corneal clouding, coarse features, growth and mental retardation. Hunter: Deficiency of L-idurano-sulfate sulfatase, coarse facies, clear cornea, growth and mental retardation
Morquio; Scheie; Maroteaux-Lamy	Aortic regurgitation	Morquio: Deficiency of N-acetylhexosamine sulfate sulfatase, cloudy cornea, severe bone changes involving vertebrae and epiphyses. Scheie: Deficiency of α-L-iduronidase, cloudy cornea, normal intelligence, peculiar facies. Maroteaux-Lamy: Deficiency of arylsulfatase B, cloudy cornea, osseous changes

Chromosomal Abnormalities

Condition	Cardiac findings	Features
Trisomy 21 (Down syndrome)	Endocardial cushion defect, atrial or ventricular septal defect, tetralogy of Fallot	Hypotonia, hyperextensible joints, mongoloid facies, mental retardation
Trisomy 13(D)	Ventricular septal defect, right ventricle patent ductus arteriosus, double-outlet right ventricle	Single midline intracerebral ventricle with midfacial defects, polydactyly, nail changes, mental retardation
Trisomy 18(E)	Congenital polyvalvular dysplasia, ventricular septal defect, patent ductus	Clenched hand, short sternum, low arch dermal ridge pattern on fingertips, mental retardation
Cri du chat (short-arm deletion-5)	Ventricular septal defect	Cat cry, microcephaly, antimongoloid slant of palpebral fissures, mental retardation
XO (Turner)	Coarctation of aorta, bicuspid aortic valve, aortic dilatation	Short female, broad chest, lymphedema, webbed neck
XXXY and XXXXX	Patent ductus arteriosus	XXXY: Hypogenitalism, mental retardation, radial-ulnar synostosis. XXXXX: Small hands, incurving of fifth fingers, mental retardation

Continued

TABLE 3-2—cont'd

Syndrome	Major Cardiovascular Manifestations	Major Noncardiac Abnormalities
Sporadic Disorders		
VATER association	Ventricular septal defect	Vertebral anomalies, anal atresia, tracheoesophageal fistula, radial and renal anomalies
CHARGE association	Tetralogy of Fallot (other defects common)	Colobomas, choanal atresia, mental and growth deficiency, genital and ear anomalies
Cornelia de Lange	Ventricular septal defect	Micromelia, synophrys, mental and growth deficiency
Teratogenic Disorders		
Rubella	Patent ductus arteriosus, pulmonic valvular and/or arterial stenosis, atrial septal defect	Cataracts, deafness, microcephaly
Alcohol	Ventricular septal defect (other defects)	Microcephaly, growth and mental deficiency, short palpebral fissures, smooth philtrum, thin upper lip
Dilantin	Pulmonic stenosis, aortic stenosis, coarctation, patent ductus arteriosus	Hypertelorism, growth and mental deficiency, short phalanges, bowed upper lip
Thalidomide	Variable	Phocomelia
Lithium	Ebstein's anomaly, tricuspid atresia	None

Modified from Friedman WF, Child JS: Congenital heart disease. In Fauci A, Braunwald E, Isselbacher KJ, et al., editors: **Harrison's principles of internal medicine**, ed 14, New York, 1998, McGraw-Hill. Copyright 1998 The McGraw-Hill Companies, Inc.

TABLE 3–3. Relative Frequency of Occurrence of Cardiac Malformations at Birth

Disease	Percentage
Ventricular septal defect	30.5
Atrial septal defect	9.8
Patent ductus arteriosus	9.7
Pulmonic stenosis	6.9
Coarctation of the aorta	6.8
Aortic stenosis	6.1
Tetralogy of Fallot	5.8
Complete transposition of the great arteries	4.2
Persistent truncus arteriosus	2.2
Tricuspid atresia	1.3
All others	16.5

From Friedman WF, Silverman N: Congenital heart disease in infancy and childhood. In Braunwald E, Zipes DP, Libby P, editors: **Heart Disease,** ed 6, Philadelphia, 2001, WB Saunders. Data based on 2310 cases.

taking the pulse or listening to the chest.

Inspection

The first step is to simply observe the child. Much information can be gained from observation, especially before a child is awakened or frightened by a stethoscope.

General Appearance

The examination should begin with an overall impression of the child. Does the child seem ill, or is he or she happy and playful? The body build should be recorded as height and weight, and these numbers should be converted to percentiles and plotted on a graph (Figure 3-1). Percentiles are very important in showing the effects of surgery and intercurrent illnesses as the child is followed over the years and development is observed.

Physical Abnormalities

Any congenital malformations or external signs of chromosomal disorders should be noted, because many are associated with heart defects (see Table 3-3). For example, half of all children with Down syndrome (Figure 3-2) have congenital heart disease, mainly endocardial cushion defects (see Chapter 15) or ventricular septal defects (see Chapter 11).

Color of Skin and Mucous Membranes

Assessment of the skin is important, because it may reflect internal processes. The color of the skin is first assessed to determine whether the child is cyanotic, pale, or jaundiced.

Cyanosis, a bluish tinge to the mucous membranes or skin, is caused by the presence of excessive unoxygenated hemoglobin in the capillaries. Mild

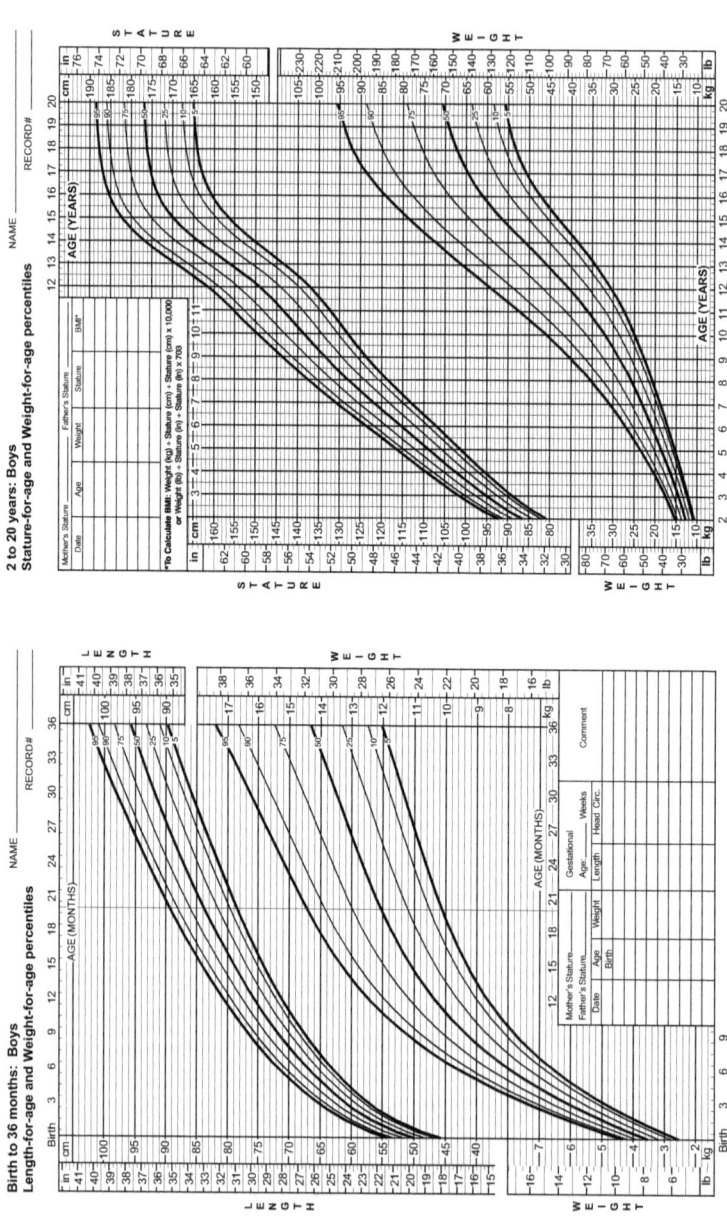

FIGURE 3-1. Charts for boys and girls of length (or stature) by age (**upper curves**) and weight by age (**lower curves**), each curve corresponding to the indicated percentile level. Note that length and stature are expressed in inches or centimeters, whereas weight is expressed in pounds or kilograms. (Developed by the National Center for Health Statistics in collaboration with the National Center for Chronic Disease Prevention and Health Promotion [2000]. http://www.cdc.gov/growthcharts)

Continued

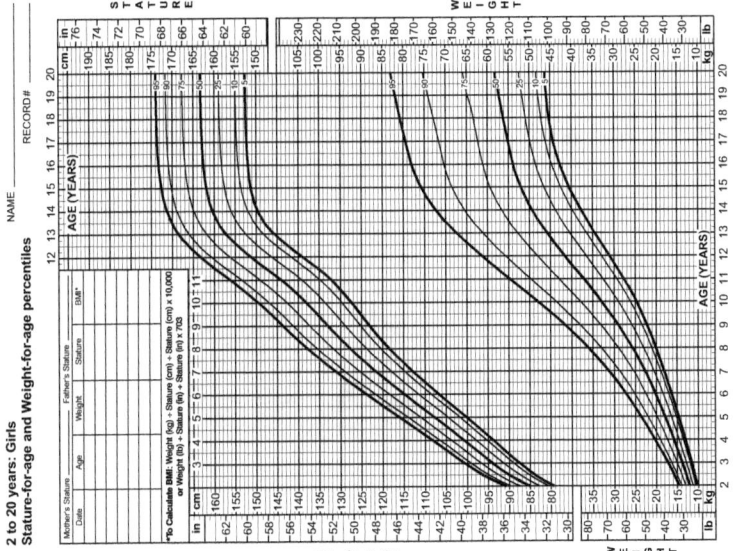

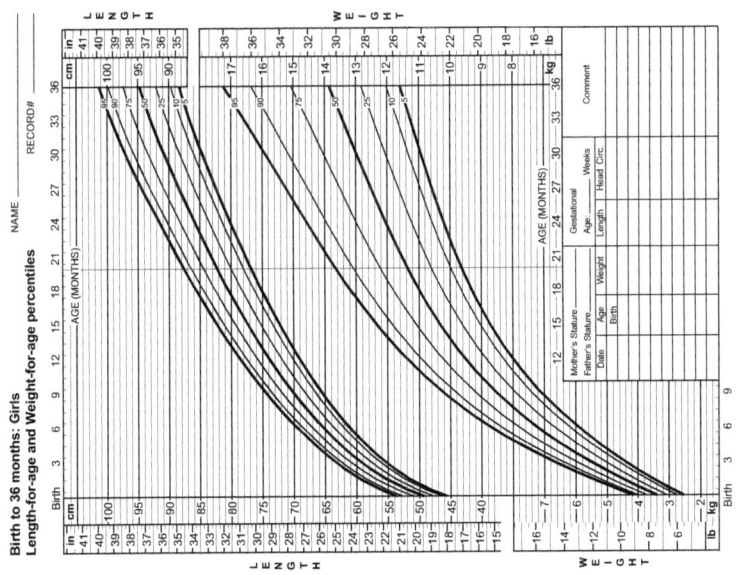

FIGURE 3-1, cont'd.

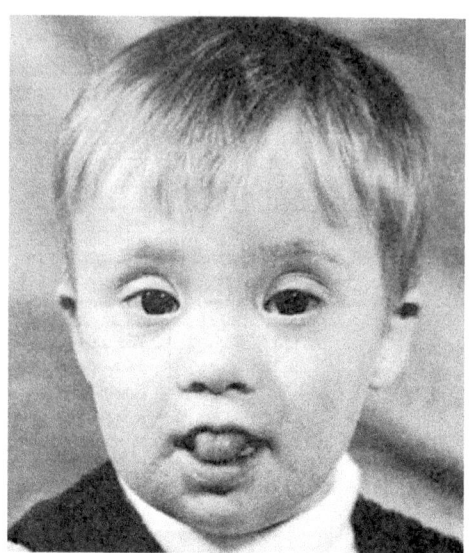

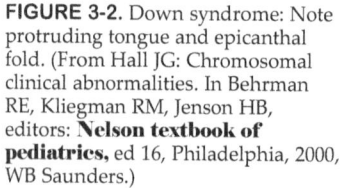

FIGURE 3-2. Down syndrome: Note protruding tongue and epicanthal fold. (From Hall JG: Chromosomal clinical abnormalities. In Behrman RE, Kliegman RM, Jenson HB, editors: **Nelson textbook of pediatrics,** ed 16, Philadelphia, 2000, WB Saunders.)

cyanosis is difficult to detect. In children with a normal hemoglobin level, arterial oxygen saturation is generally below 85% (normal is 95% to 99%) before cyanosis is visible. Cyanosis is most easily seen under natural light; it may be more difficult to see under artificial light. Cyanosis is also difficult to detect in children with deeply pigmented skin, and examination of these children must include additional structures such as the tongue, buccal mucosa, nail beds, and conjunctiva.

In addition to its presence, the distribution of the cyanosis should be recorded. Is the entire body cyanotic or just one part? Children with patent ductus arteriosus and pulmonary hypertension with right-to-left shunt may have cyanotic fingers of the left hand but not the right (see Chapter 13). Sometimes only the lower half of the body is cyanotic.

Some children with cyanosis do not have cyanotic congenital heart disease. The cyanosis may be caused by respiratory disease or abnormalities of the central nervous system. When the blood does not contain enough oxygen (arterial desaturation), the condition is called **central cyanosis.** Cyanosis associated with normal blood oxygen levels is termed **peripheral cyanosis** and is seen in two conditions in children: (1) exposure to cold and (2) congestive heart failure (the cyanosis is a consequence of sluggish peripheral blood flow). Cyanosis caused by lung disease in a newborn can often be distinguished from cyanosis resulting from cardiac disease by the hyperoxia test. In this test, the infant is given 100% oxygen to breathe. If there is little change in the cyanosis and blood oxygen concentration, the cyanosis is caused by heart disease. If lung disease is responsible, the cyanosis usually decreases in response to oxygen administration.

Even mild cyanosis in a newborn merits thorough study. Oxygen saturation can be determined noninvasively by pulse oximetry. The hematocrit level must be measured. An elevated hematocrit indicates polycythemia, an inevitable consequence of diminished oxygen level in arterial blood. The hematocrit level is an index that should be regularly monitored in children with cyanotic congenital heart disease.

Pallor may be present in infants with vasoconstriction from serious congestive heart failure or shock as well as in cases of severe anemia.

Jaundice, a yellowish discoloration of the skin, may be caused by congenital hypothyroidism associated with patent ductus arteriosus and pulmonic valve stenosis. However, jaundice very rarely has any relationship to heart disease.

Clubbing

The fingers should be examined for clubbing. In its early stages, clubbing can be detected by noting whether the normal slight angle is present between the nail and the nail bed (Figure 3-3). This angle is lost in early clubbing, and the base of the nail bed feels soft and spongy. As clubbing progresses, the nail feels as though it is floating in a bed of soft vascular tissue. In advanced clubbing, the nail assumes a so-called **watch glass deformity,** and the fingertips become wider and rounder. The overlying skin stretches, loses normal wrinkles, and has a polished, glistening appearance.

Low arterial oxygen levels of long duration, generally more than 6 months, produce clubbing of the fingers and toes, even when the associated cyanosis is too mild to be seen. Other disorders that produce clubbing include lung disease, especially an abscess; cirrhosis of the liver; and subacute bacterial endocarditis. Some normal individuals may also be affected, a condition called **familial clubbing.**

Respiration

The respiratory rate of every infant and child should be assessed and recorded. If breathing is irregular, the rate should be counted for a full minute. Respiratory rate is most reliably assessed during sleep. The rate is increased in children who are crying, upset, eating, or febrile. After feeding, an infant may breathe more rapidly for as long as 5 or 10 minutes. A respiratory rate of 40 breaths per minute is normal for an infant but abnormal for an older child. A rate of more than 60 breaths per minute is abnormal even in a newborn. Rapid breathing and rapid heartbeat are early signs of left ventricular failure, especially if there are no other signs of distress (effortless tachypnea). Breathing that is rapid and labored may be caused by lung disease.

Observation of the Chest

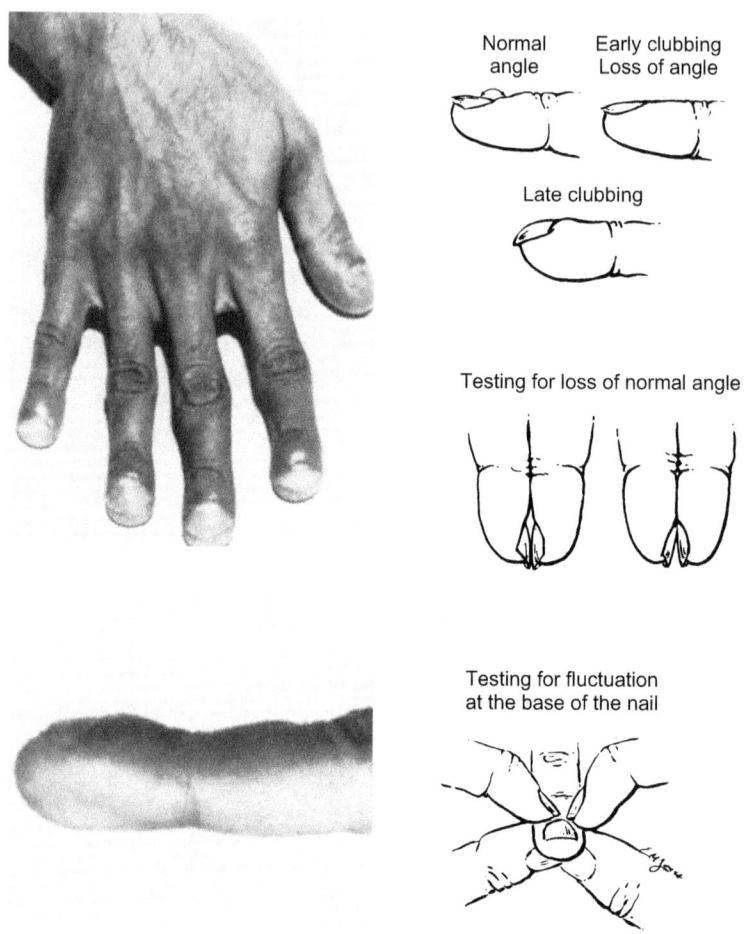

Normal angle   Early clubbing
                Loss of angle

Late clubbing

Testing for loss of normal angle

Testing for fluctuation
at the base of the nail

FIGURE 3-3. Left, Top view of the right-hand and side view of the index finger of a patient with advanced clubbing resulting from interstitial lung disease. **Right,** Signs of and tests for clubbing. (**Left,** from Hinshaw HC, Murray JF: **Diseases of the chest,** ed 4, Philadelphia, 1980, WB Saunders. **Right,** from Lehrer S: **Understanding lung sounds,** ed 3, Philadelphia, 2001, WB Saunders.)

Inspection of the chest begins with noting any deformities. The precordium (the region over the heart) is assessed for bulging and pulsations, which may suggest chronic cardiac enlargement. **Pectus excavatum,** or **funnel chest** (Figure 3-4), rarely interferes with heart function but may cause a pulmonary systolic ejection murmur (see Chapter 11) or a large heart shadow on the chest x-ray film. **Pectus carinatum,** or **pigeon chest,** may be associated with Marfan syndrome. Visible pulsations, sometimes rocking

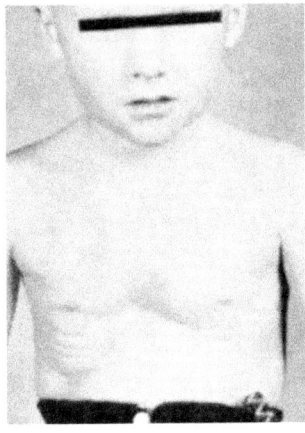 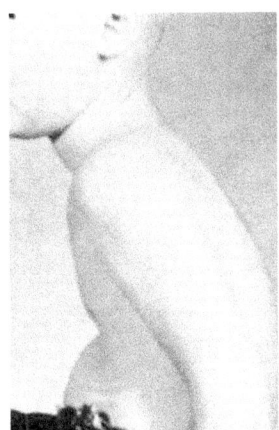

FIGURE 3-4. Pectus excavatum (funnel chest) in a 4-year-old boy. Note the rounded shoulders, kyphosis (hunchback), and protuberant abdomen. (From Salzberg AM: Congenital malformations of the lower respiratory tract. In Kendig EL, Chernick V, editors: **Disorders of the respiratory tract of children,** ed 4, Philadelphia, 1983, WB Saunders.)

the whole chest, are occasionally seen in patients with congenital heart disease and tremendous shunts or in children with aortic or mitral regurgitation. **Harrison's groove,** a depressed line along the bottom of the rib cage where the diaphragm attaches, indicates stiff lungs (poor pulmonary compliance) and is present in children with large left-to-right shunts (Figure 3-5). Retraction of the skin between the ribs and in the sternal notch on inspiration is a sign of respiratory distress. The left side of the chest may be prominent because of increased heart size.

Other Observations

Infants with congestive heart failure often have a cold sweat on the forehead; their diminished cardiac output causes compensatory overactivity of the sympathetic nervous system, which controls sweating. Vigorous arterial pulsation in the neck can be seen in children with aortic defects such as coarctation of the aorta, patent ductus arteriosus, or aortic regurgitation. A crude estimate of venous pressure can be made in an older child by observing the jugular vein. If the child is recumbent, the height of the blood column in the vein should not rise above an imaginary straight line across the manubrium of the sternum (Figure 3-6). Elevated jugular venous pressure is a sign of right heart failure.

Palpation

Palpation is generally the next step after inspection. If an infant is sleeping, it may be more productive to skip to auscultation (discussed later), because palpation might cause the infant to awaken, cry, and become uncooperative.

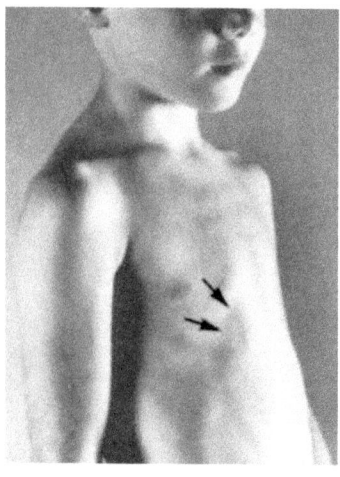
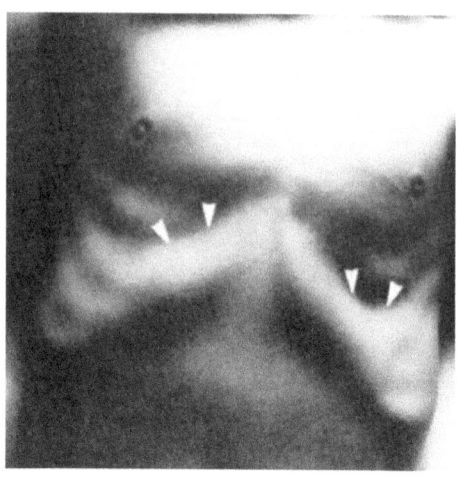

A   B

FIGURE 3-5. A, Five-year-old boy with a large shunt through an ostium secundum atrial septal defect. The child's physical appearance is delicate, frail, and gracile. Weight has been affected but height has not. A shallow pectus excavatum is evident. Harrison's grooves are identified by the **arrows. B,** Six-year-old girl with a large shunt through an ostium secundum atrial septal defect. Lighting was arranged to emphasize Harrison's grooves **(arrowheads).** (From Perloff JK: **The clinical recognition of congenital heart disease,** ed 4, Philadelphia, 1994, WB Saunders.)

FIGURE 3-6. A crude estimate of venous pressure in an older child can be obtained by observing the jugular vein. If the child is recumbent, the tip of the blood column in the vein **(ZL)** should not rise above an imaginary straight line across the manubrium line **(ML)** of the sternum. Note that the child is lying at a 45-degree angle. (From Nadas AS, Fyler DC: **Pediatric cardiology,** ed 3, Philadelphia, 1972, WB Saunders. Copyright AS Nadas.)

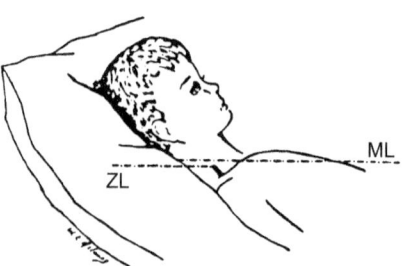

Peripheral Pulses

The pulse rate should be counted and any irregularities noted. The pulse rate diminishes with age (Table 3-4) and is affected by the patient's condition. **Tachycardia** (an increased pulse rate) is found in children with fever, congestive heart failure, or arrhythmia or in a child who is excited. **Bradycardia** (a slow pulse rate) can be caused by heart block, digitalis toxicity, or (in an older, athletic child) by vigorous physical conditioning. An irregular pulse may occur because of an abnormality of the conduction system. Notably, sinus arrhythmia, an acceleration of the pulse with inspiration, is normal.

A comparison should be made between the forcefulness of the pulse in

TABLE 3–4. Average Pulse Rates at Rest

Age	Lower Limits of Normal		Average		Upper Limits of Normal	
Newborn	70/min		125/min		190/min	
1-11 months	80		120		160	
2 years	80		110		130	
4 years	80		100		120	
6 years	75		100		115	
8 years	70		90		110	
10 years	70		90		110	
	Girls	**Boys**	**Girls**	**Boys**	**Girls**	**Boys**
12 years	70	65	90	85	110	105
14 years	65	60	85	80	105	100
16 years	60	55	80	75	100	95
18 years	55	50	75	70	95	90

From Behrman R, Vaughan VC: **Nelson textbook of pediatrics,** ed 12, Philadelphia, 1983, WB Saunders.

the right and left arms, and also in an arm and a leg (Figures 3-7 and 3-8). The dorsalis pedis or posterior tibial pulses (Figure 3-9) may be preferable to the femoral pulse, because attempts to palpate the femoral pulses sometimes awaken a sleeping infant or upset a toddler.

If the leg pulses are much weaker than the arm pulses, coarctation of the aorta may be present (Figure 3-10). If the dorsalis pedis or posterior tibial pulses are strong, the presence of coarctation is unlikely. If the right brachial pulse is stronger than the left, the aorta may be narrowed near the origin of the left subclavian artery. If any doubt exists about the strength of distal lower extremity pulses, the simultaneity of radial and femoral pulses should be assessed to rule out aortic coarctation.

A **bounding pulse** is associated with patent ductus arteriosus, aortic insufficiency, a large arteriovenous fistula, or, rarely, persistent truncus arteriosus (a defect in which a large single vessel arises from the heart, dividing into the coronary and pulmonary arteries and the aortic arch with its usual branches). Pulses are often bounding in premature infants because of lack of subcutaneous tissue and because many have patent ductus arteriosus. Bounding pulses are also present in children treated for cyanotic congenital heart lesions with large, surgically created systemic-pulmonary shunts (see Chapter 14).

Pulses that are weak and thready may be found in cardiac failure, circulatory shock, or severe aortic stenosis and hypoplastic left ventricle syndrome. A weak pulse may also be found in the leg of a child with coarctation of the aorta. An absent or weak radial pulse is found in children after surgical construction of systemic-pulmonary shunts involving the subclavian artery on the side of the shunt (Blalock-Taussig procedure; see Chapter 14).

Pulsus paradoxus (paradoxical pulsation) is characterized by an excessive variation in the forcefulness of the arterial pulsation during the

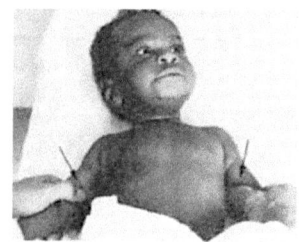

FIGURE 3-7. Comparison of the right and left brachial arterial pulses **(arrows)** by simultaneous palpation. (From Perloff JK: **Physical examination of the heart and circulation,** ed 3, Philadelphia, 2000, WB Saunders.)

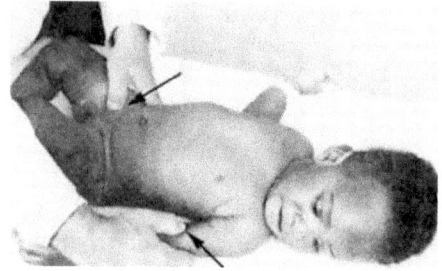

FIGURE 3-8. Comparison of femoral and brachial arterial pulses by simultaneous palpation **(arrows).** (From Perloff JK: **Physical examination of the heart and circulation,** ed 3, Philadelphia, 2000, WB Saunders.)

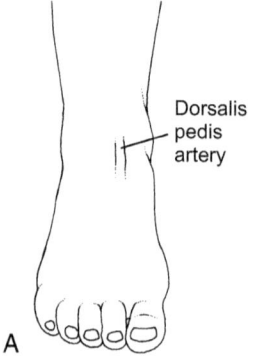

Dorsalis pedis artery

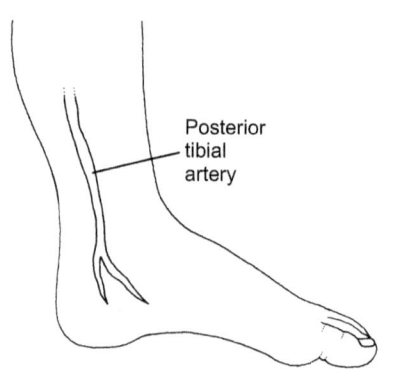

Posterior tibial artery

A   B

FIGURE 3-9. Location of the dorsalis pedis **(A)** and posterior tibial **(B)** pulses.

respiratory cycle. During inspiration there is normally a reduction in systolic pressure of a few millimeters of mercury. If the reduction is more than 10 mm Hg, pulsus paradoxus is said to exist. Despite its name, pulsus paradoxus is not a phase reversal of the pulse pressure variation during respiration. One cause of pulsus paradoxus is cardiac tamponade resulting from pericardial effusion. The abnormal fluid collection filling the pericardial sac, which encases the heart, causes excessive compression and interferes with cardiac function, especially during inspiration. Constrictive pericarditis (rare in children), which has the same functional end result, also produces pulsus paradoxus. Very rarely, pulsus paradoxus is seen in

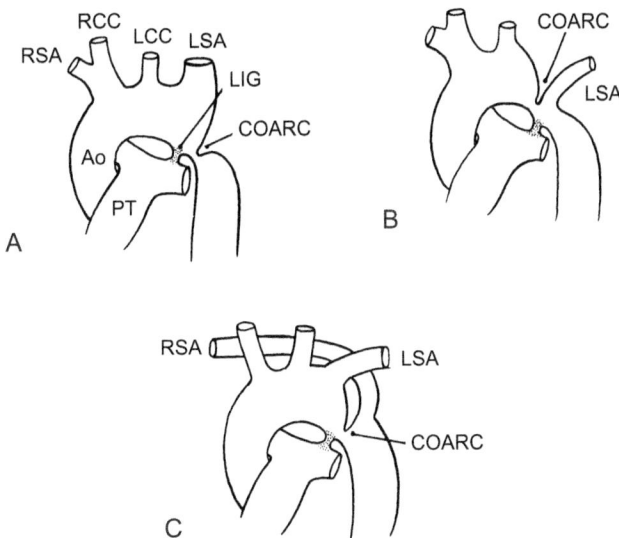

FIGURE 3-10. Illustrations of the typical variety of coarctation (**COARC**) of the aorta and two anatomic variations. **A,** In the typical variety, the coarctation is located immediately beyond the left subclavian artery (**LSA**), which is enlarged. The descending aorta is dilated distal to the coarctation. **B,** The site of coarctation is just proximal to the left subclavian artery. The left subclavian artery is not dilated. **C,** The right subclavian artery (**RSA**) arises anomalously below the coarctation. **Ao,** Ascending aorta; **LCC,** left common carotid artery; **LIG,** ligamentum arteriosum; **PT,** pulmonary trunk; **RCC,** right common carotid artery; **RSA,** right subclavian artery. (From Perloff JK: **The clinical recognition of congenital heart disease,** ed 4, Philadelphia, 1994, WB Saunders.)

children with severe respiratory distress caused by asthma or pneumonia. Instructions for precise assessment of pulsus paradoxus are given in the section on blood pressure determination.

Chest

Palpation of the chest includes the following determinations: the apical impulse, the point of maximum impulse, hyperactivity of the precordium, and precordial thrill.

Apical Impulse. Palpation of the apical impulse may help in the detection of cardiomegaly (enlargement of the heart). Although percussion (tapping on the chest to elicit dullness over the area of the heart) may be of help in identifying cardiomegaly in adults, it is of less value in children, and palpation is more important. Both the location and quality of the apical impulse should be determined by palpation. After the age of 7 years the apical impulse is normally located at the fifth intercostal space in the midclavicular line (Figure 3-11). Before this age, the apical impulse occurs in the fourth intercostal space just to the left of the midclavicular line. Any downward or lateral displacement of the apical impulse may indicate enlargement of the heart.

Point of Maximum Impulse. Locating the point of maximum impulse (PMI) aids in determining whether the right or left ventricle is dominant. If the right ventricle is dominant, the impulse is maximal at the lower left sternal border. If the left ventricle is dominant, the impulse is maximal at the apex. Normal newborns and infants have more right ventricular dominance and right ventricular impulse than older children. A diffuse, gradually rising impulse is called a **heave** and usually indicates a volume overload of the heart. A sharply localized, quickly rising impulse is called a **tap** and usually implies a pressure overload.

Hyperactivity of the Precordium. The precordium appears quite active in two classes of heart disease:

1. Cases of volume overload present in congenital heart disease with

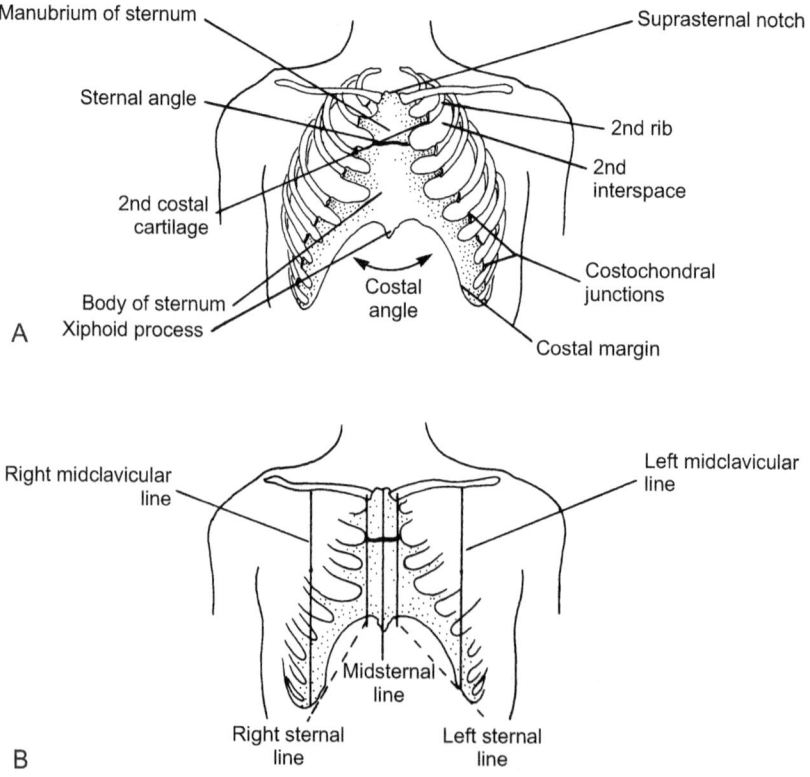

FIGURE 3-11. A, Anatomy of the chest wall. Reference lines on the chest wall: **B,** Anterior view.

Continued

large left-to-right shunts, such as patent ductus arteriosus or ventricular septal defect

2. Cases of severe valvular insufficiency, such as aortic or mitral insufficiency

Precordial Thrill. A thrill is a fine vibration felt by the hand and corresponds to the sound of a murmur heard through the stethoscope. Thrills are best detected with the palm of the hand, rather than the finger-

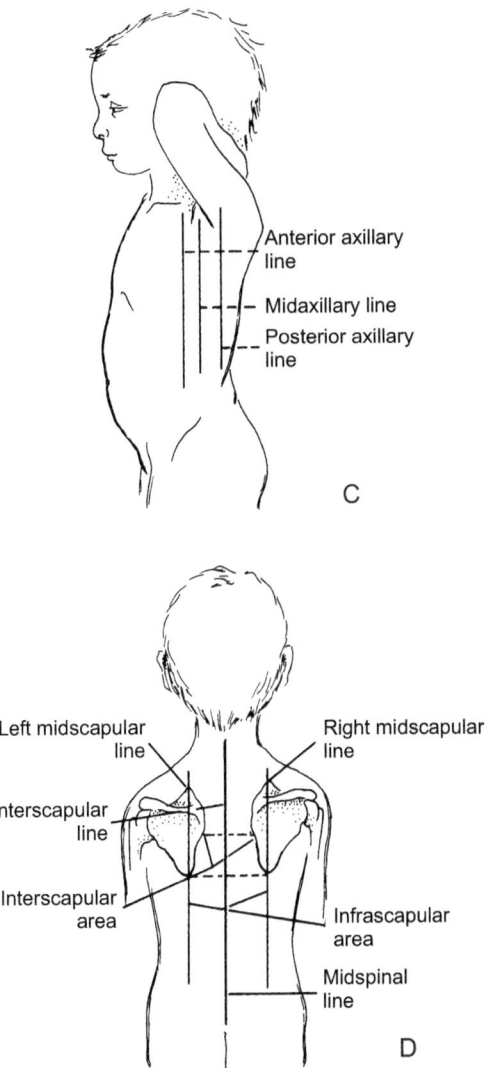

FIGURE 3-11, cont'd. **C,** axillary view, and **D,** posterior view.

tips, although the fingertips are needed to feel a thrill in the suprasternal notch or over the carotid arteries. The location of a thrill may be of diagnostic value in the following instances:

1. A thrill over the upper left sternal border is generated by the pulmonary artery or pulmonic valve and occurs in pulmonary valvular stenosis, pulmonary arterial stenosis, or, occasionally, patent ductus arteriosus.
2. A thrill over the upper right sternal border is often of aortic origin and may indicate aortic stenosis.
3. A thrill over the lower left sternal border is associated with ventricular septal defects.
4. A thrill in the suprasternal notch may be caused by aortic stenosis but is also found in pulmonic valve stenosis and patent ductus arteriosus. Coarctation of the aorta does not usually cause a thrill in the suprasternal notch unless aortic stenosis is also present.
5. A thrill over one or both carotid arteries, accompanied by a thrill in the suprasternal notch, may result from a deformity of the aorta (for example, coarctation) or of the aortic valve (for example, aortic stenosis). A thrill in a single carotid artery may be a **bruit** (from the French for "noise") originating in the carotid itself.
6. In an older child, a thrill in one or more left intercostal spaces may indicate coarctation of the aorta and extensive intercostal collaterals (Figure 3-12).

Abdomen

Palpation of the abdomen is an important step in the examination of the child with cardiac disease because congestive heart failure produces significant changes in the liver. The most important determination is locating the liver edge. In normal infants and young children, the edge may be as far as 2 cm below the right costal margin in the midclavicular line. When assessing for the liver position, the clinician should try not to irritate the child. The abdomen should be palpated very gently while the examiner feels for the right lobe of the liver. Sometimes, to determine the approximate site of the liver edge, initial percussion of the abdomen over the liver is helpful. Percussion usually does not perturb the child and increases the chance of feeling the edge before the child becomes agitated.

Daily observation of liver size is a reliable guide for assessing the degree of congestive failure in a child. In severe congestive failure, the liver edge may be palpable 7 cm below the right costal margin. After failure has been adequately treated, the edge may no longer be palpable. Besides being enlarged, the liver in congestive failure may be tender and usually has a less well-defined edge. Another sign of congenital heart disease is a pulsatile liver. This sign can be found in children with tricuspid regurgitation or severe pulmonic valve stenosis.

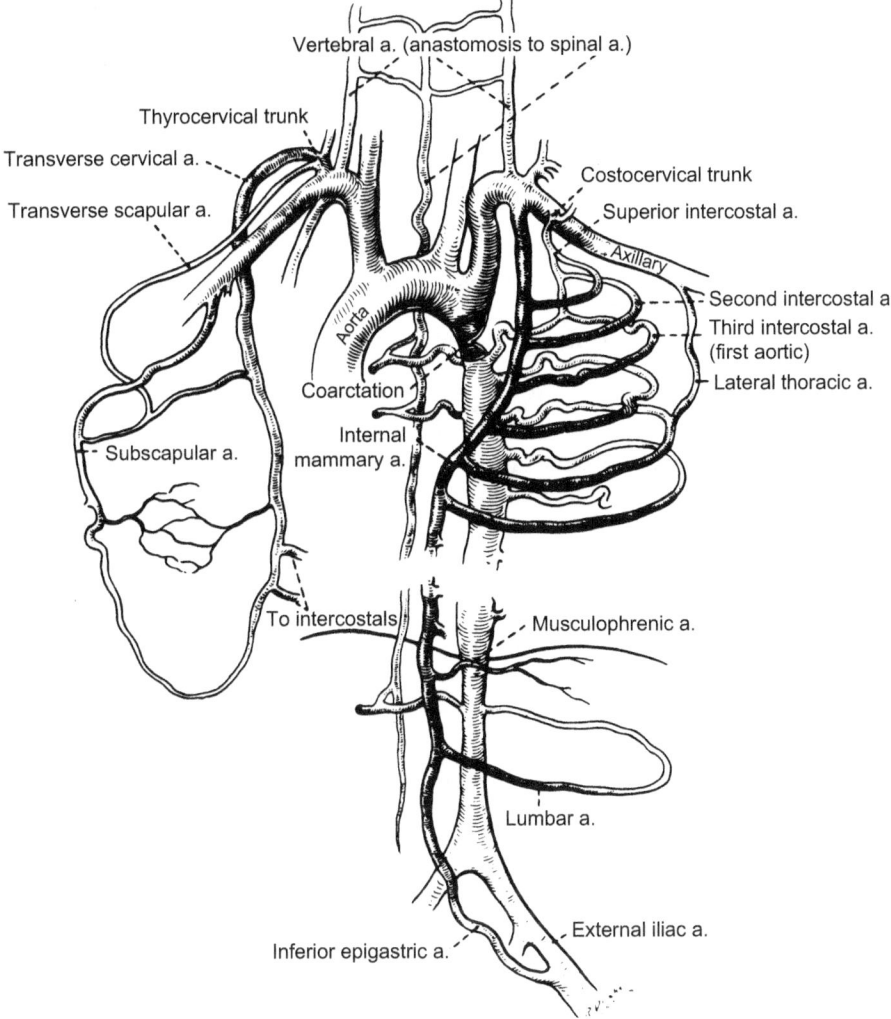

FIGURE 3-12. Collateral circulation in coarctation of the aorta. **a,** Artery. (From Edwards JE, Clagett OT, Drake RL et al: The collateral circulation in coarctation of the aorta, **Mayo Clin Proc** 23:333, 1948.)

Although many young children normally have a palpable spleen, an enlarged spleen is a hallmark of bacterial endocarditis and should be investigated. Congestive heart failure seldom causes splenic enlargement. Malposition of the spleen and liver, in which the spleen is on the right side and the liver is on the left (abdominal situs inversus), may be associated with congenital heart disease.

BLOOD PRESSURE DETERMINATION

Blood pressure determination is an integral part of every examination. Blood pressure should be measured not only in the arms but also in the legs, because, as was mentioned, a marked difference may be caused by coarctation of the aorta. The auscultatory method of blood pressure determination, using a mercury sphygmomanometer, is easy and tolerated well by older children. Assessment of blood pressure in younger children is more difficult because (1) the child may be uncooperative, (2) limbs of different sizes require different cuff widths, and (3) results must be interpreted with regard to the age of the child (Tables 3-5 and 3-6).

The child is most likely to cooperate if the procedure is explained beforehand. Pointing out the fluctuations of the mercury column, for example, may help to distract the older child. A pacifier or bottle may help to calm an infant.

Cuff size is critical if auscultatory results are to be comparable with those obtained by direct arterial puncture. The cuff should cover three fourths of the upper arm or leg. A cuff that is too narrow gives falsely high readings, and a large cuff may yield low readings. Therefore, 3-, 5-, 7-, 12-, and 18-cm cuffs should be available. The examiner must also select a cuff of the proper length. The bladder must be 20% to 25% longer than the average circumference of the limb. This standard is recommended by the American Heart Association for adults and applies equally to children. A short cuff gives falsely high blood pressure readings for obese children, because it does not adequately encircle the limb.

After applying a cuff of the proper size, the examiner should obtain a preliminary estimate of the systolic pressure by palpation. First the cuff is inflated to a point well above the obliteration of the pulse in the antecubital fossa. Then gradually, 1 to 3 mm Hg per heartbeat, the pressure should be released until the pulse reappears. This point corresponds closely with the systolic pressure as assessed by direct arterial puncture.

In auscultatory measurement of blood pressure, a series of sounds **(Korotkoff sounds)** are identified and correlated with pressure readings on the manometer. The first step is to locate by palpation the brachial artery in the antecubital fossa (Figure 3-13). The diaphragm of the stethoscope should be placed directly over the artery. The cuff is then inflated as quickly as possible to a point above the systolic pressure. The systolic pressure corresponds to the mercury level at which the first Korotkoff sound is audible.

The Korotkoff sounds may be divided into five phases: (1) a tapping sound, (2) a softening of the tapping sound, (3) a murmur, (4) a muffling of the sound, and (5) a disappearance of the sound. To obtain this sequence in an uninterrupted manner, rapid inflation of the cuff is essential. If the cuff is inflated too slowly, an auscultatory gap appears. An auscultatory gap means that the sounds become inaudible, then audible again. The auscultatory gap may cause an erroneously low estimation of systolic pressure.

TABLE 3–5. Blood Pressure Levels for the 90th and 95th Percentiles of Blood Pressure for Boys Aged 1 to 17 Years by Percentiles of Height

Age (yr)	Blood Pressure Percentile*	Systolic Blood Pressure by Percentile of Height (mm Hg)†							Diastolic Blood Pressure by Percentile of Height (mm Hg)†						
		5%	10%	25%	50%	75%	90%	95%	5%	10%	25%	50%	75%	90%	95%
1	90th	94	95	97	98	100	102	102	50	51	52	53	54	54	55
	95th	98	99	101	102	104	106	106	55	55	56	57	58	59	59
2	90th	98	99	100	102	104	105	106	55	55	56	57	58	59	59
	95th	101	102	104	106	108	109	110	59	59	60	61	62	63	63
3	90th	100	101	103	105	107	108	109	59	59	60	61	62	63	63
	95th	104	105	107	109	111	112	113	63	63	64	65	66	67	67
4	90th	102	103	105	107	109	110	111	62	62	63	64	65	66	66
	95th	106	107	109	111	113	114	115	66	67	67	68	69	70	71
5	90th	104	105	106	108	110	112	112	65	65	66	67	68	69	69
	95th	108	109	110	112	114	115	116	69	70	70	71	72	73	74
6	90th	105	106	108	110	111	113	114	67	68	69	70	70	71	72
	95th	109	110	112	114	115	117	117	72	72	73	74	75	76	76
7	90th	106	107	109	111	113	114	115	69	70	71	72	72	73	74
	95th	110	111	113	115	116	118	119	74	74	75	76	77	78	78
8	90th	107	108	110	112	114	115	116	71	71	72	73	74	75	75
	95th	111	112	114	116	118	119	120	75	76	76	77	78	79	80
9	90th	109	110	112	113	115	117	117	72	73	73	74	75	76	77
	95th	113	114	116	117	119	121	121	76	77	78	79	80	80	81
10	90th	110	112	113	115	117	118	119	73	74	74	75	76	77	78
	95th	114	115	117	119	121	122	123	77	78	79	80	80	81	82
11	90th	112	113	115	117	119	120	121	74	74	75	76	77	78	78
	95th	116	117	119	121	123	124	125	78	78	79	80	81	82	82
12	90th	115	116	117	119	121	123	123	75	75	76	77	78	78	79
	95th	119	120	121	123	125	126	127	79	79	80	81	82	82	83
13	90th	117	118	120	122	124	125	126	75	76	76	77	78	79	80
	95th	121	122	124	126	128	129	130	79	80	81	82	83	83	83
14	90th	120	121	123	125	126	128	128	76	76	77	78	79	79	80
	95th	124	125	127	128	130	132	132	80	81	81	82	83	84	84
15	90th	123	124	125	127	129	131	131	77	77	78	79	80	81	81
	95th	127	128	129	131	133	134	135	81	82	83	83	84	85	86
16	90th	125	126	128	130	132	133	134	79	79	80	81	82	82	83
	95th	129	130	132	134	136	137	138	83	83	84	85	86	87	87
17	90th	128	129	131	133	134	136	136	81	81	82	83	84	85	85
	95th	132	133	135	136	138	140	140	85	85	86	87	88	89	89

From Seidel H et al: **Mosby's guide to physical examination**, ed 4, St Louis, 1999, Mosby.
Data from Update on the Task Force Report (1987) on High Blood Pressure in Children and Adolescents: A working group report from National High Blood Pressure Education Program, NIH 96-3790.
Printed in Update on Task Force Report on High Blood Pressure in Children, **Pediatrics** 98:649-658, 1996.
*Blood pressure percentile was determined by a single measurement.
†Height percentile was determined by standard growth curves.

TABLE 3–6. Blood Pressure Levels for the 90th and 95th Percentiles of Blood Pressure for Girls Aged 1 to 17 Years by Percentiles of Height

Age (yr)	Blood Pressure Percentile*	Systolic Blood Pressure by Percentile of Height (mm Hg)†							Diastolic Blood Pressure by Percentile of Height (mm Hg)†						
		5%	10%	25%	50%	75%	90%	95%	5%	10%	25%	50%	75%	90%	95%
1	90th	97	98	99	100	102	103	104	53	53	53	54	55	56	56
	95th	101	102	103	104	105	107	107	57	57	57	58	59	60	60
2	90th	99	99	10	102	103	104	105	57	57	58	58	59	60	61
	95th	102	103	104	105	107	108	109	61	61	62	62	63	64	65
3	90th	100	100	102	103	104	105	106	61	61	61	62	63	63	64
	95th	104	104	105	107	108	109	110	65	65	65	66	67	67	68
4	90th	101	102	103	104	106	107	108	63	63	64	65	65	66	67
	95th	105	106	107	108	109	111	111	67	67	68	69	69	70	71
5	90th	103	103	104	106	107	108	109	65	66	66	67	68	68	69
	95th	107	107	108	110	111	112	113	69	70	70	71	72	72	73
6	90th	104	105	106	107	109	110	111	67	67	68	69	69	70	71
	95th	108	109	110	111	112	114	114	71	71	72	73	73	74	75
7	90th	106	107	108	109	110	112	112	69	69	69	70	71	72	72
	95th	110	110	112	113	114	115	116	73	73	73	74	75	76	76
8	90th	108	109	110	111	112	113	114	70	70	71	71	72	73	74
	95th	112	112	113	115	116	117	118	74	74	75	75	76	77	78
9	90th	110	110	112	113	114	115	116	71	72	72	73	74	74	75
	95th	114	114	115	117	118	119	120	75	76	76	77	78	78	79
10	90th	112	112	114	115	116	117	118	73	73	73	74	75	76	76
	95th	116	116	117	119	120	121	122	77	77	77	78	79	80	80
11	90th	114	114	116	117	118	119	120	74	74	75	75	76	77	77
	95th	118	118	119	121	122	123	124	78	78	79	79	80	81	81
12	90th	116	116	118	119	120	121	122	75	75	76	76	77	78	78
	95th	120	120	121	123	124	125	126	79	79	80	80	81	82	82
13	90th	118	118	119	121	122	123	124	76	76	77	78	78	79	80
	95th	121	122	123	125	126	127	128	80	80	81	82	82	83	84
14	90th	119	120	121	122	124	125	126	77	77	78	79	79	80	81
	95th	123	124	125	126	128	129	130	81	81	82	83	83	84	85
15	90th	121	121	122	124	125	126	127	78	78	79	79	80	81	82
	95th	124	125	126	128	129	130	131	82	82	83	83	84	85	86
16	90th	122	122	123	125	126	127	128	79	79	79	80	81	82	82
	95th	125	126	127	128	130	131	132	83	83	83	84	85	86	86
17	90th	122	123	124	125	126	128	128	79	79	79	80	81	82	82
	95th	126	126	127	129	130	131	132	83	83	83	84	85	86	86

From Seidel et al: **Mosby's guide to physical examination**, ed 4, St Louis, 1999, Mosby.
Data from Uptake on the Task Force Report (1987) on High Blood Pressure in Children and Adolescents: A working group report from National High Blood Pressure Education Program, NIH 96-3790.
Printed in Update on Task Force Report for High Blood Pressure in Children, **Pediatrics** 98:649-658, 1995.
*Blood pressure percentile was determined by a single measurement.
†Height percentile was determined by standard growth curves.

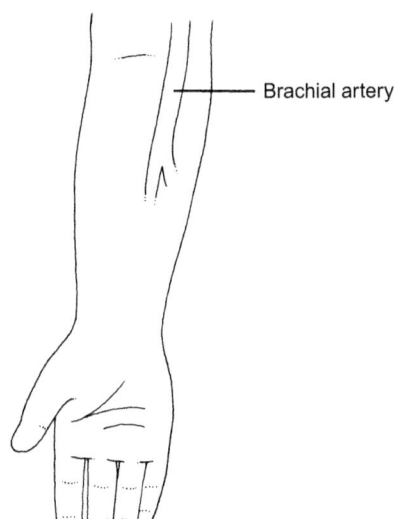

— Brachial artery

FIGURE 3-13. Location of brachial artery in antecubital fossa.

Although there is agreement that systolic pressure be considered the point at which the tapping sound is heard (phase 1), there is still some confusion as to which Korotkoff phase, 4 or 5, corresponds to the diastolic pressure in children. Some clinicians contend that phase 4, the point of muffling, is closer to the true diastolic pressure than phase 5, the point of disappearance. Therefore, when the points of muffling and disappearance are more than 6 mm Hg apart, both values should be recorded. A blood pressure of 105/70-50, for example, indicates that the systolic pressure is 105 mm Hg (the reading at phase 1 of the Korotkoff sounds), that 70 mm Hg is the reading at the point of muffling, and that 50 mm Hg is the reading at the point of disappearance. If the points of muffling and disappearance are separated by less than 6 mm, the point of disappearance is generally recorded as the diastolic pressure.

The specific procedure for measuring blood pressure in the assessment of pulsus paradoxus is outlined below. The procedure requires a very cooperative patient and is rarely possible in a young child. Specific steps in assessment of pulsus paradoxus include the following:

1. Raise the cuff pressure 20 mm Hg above the systolic pressure.
2. Reduce the pressure slowly until the phase 1 Korotkoff sound is audible for some but not all beats. Record the pressure at this point (Figure 3-14, line A).
3. Reduce the cuff pressure further until systolic sounds are audible for all beats; again, record the pressure (Figure 3-14, line B).
4. If there is more than a 10 mm Hg difference between readings A and B, pulsus paradoxus is present.

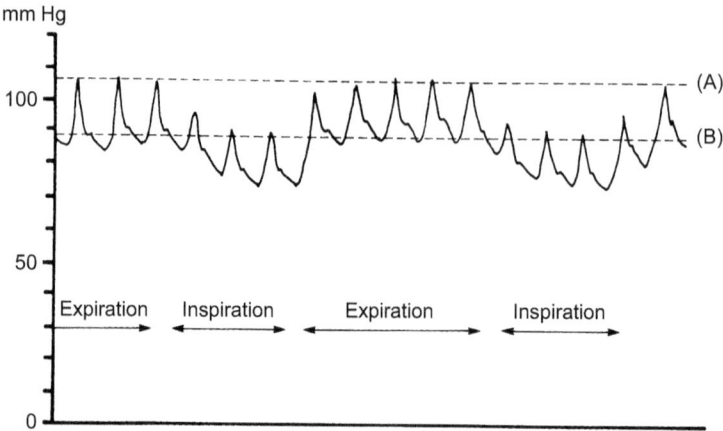

FIGURE 3-14. Diagram of pulsus paradoxus. Note the reduction of systolic pressure of more than 10 mm Hg during inspiration. (From Park MK: **Pediatric cardiology for practitioners,** ed 3, St Louis, 1996, Mosby.)

The **flush technique** is sometimes used to assess systolic blood pressure in an infant. The proper-sized cuff is placed around the infant's forearm or calf. If the forearm is used, it should be elevated and the hand grasped firmly so that as large an area as possible is blanched. The pressure applied should be sufficient to cause blanching but not to make the infant cry. The pressure is maintained while the cuff pressure is elevated. The cuff is then slowly deflated, and the hand is watched closely for signs of flushing. The point at which the flush first appears in the blanched area is taken as the systolic blood pressure. Although the flush technique is easy and relatively reliable, it has the following disadvantages:

1. It may be difficult to recognize the first sign of flushing in a cyanotic baby.
2. The pressure reading may be affected by the rapidity with which the cuff is deflated.
3. The pressure reading is more likely to be a mean pressure than a true systolic pressure.
4. In an infant with coarctation of the aorta, but not a large difference between pressure in the arm and leg, it may be difficult to demonstrate any pressure difference at all with the flush technique, especially if early heart failure is present.

Because of the difficulties in obtaining accurate blood pressure readings in either very young or very ill babies, the Dinamap, an automatic, noninvasive blood pressure monitor using oscillometric measurement, is employed in many hospital nurseries and intensive care units.

ADDITIONAL DIAGNOSTIC METHODS
Oximetry

To detect cyanosis, clinicians may use an ear oximeter to measure blood oxygen saturation. In children with dark skin this measurement is especially important, because cyanosis may not be readily visible. To assess oxygen saturation over the long term, the clinician follows the hematocrit and hemoglobin levels and red blood cell count, which rise when the blood is poorly oxygenated. Repeated oximetry measurements on successive office visits are also helpful.

Chest X-ray Studies

A chest x-ray evaluation shows whether the heart is normal in size or enlarged. Thus in a child who is breathing rapidly, the chest x-ray film can indicate whether the heart is normal or whether heart failure is present. In addition, certain heart lesions have a characteristic cardiac silhouette. For example, in tetralogy of Fallot, the heart is normal in size but boot shaped, with an elevated apex and a small or concave pulmonary segment. In "corrected" transposition of the great arteries (L-transposition), the aorta creates a characteristically convex "shoulder" where the pulmonary artery normally lies. Chest x-ray studies are also useful for assessing pulmonary flow and pulmonary vasculature and indicate whether pulmonary vasculature is normal, increased, or decreased. Increased pulmonary vasculature suggests a left-to-right shunt or pulmonary venous obstruction. Decreased pulmonary vasculature suggests a right-to-left shunt.

Two-Dimensional Echocardiography

Two-dimensional echocardiography, which uses reflected sound waves, was developed from the same technology used for sonar detection of submarines. Echocardiography is the most common method for confirming a diagnosis of congenital heart disease. The echocardiogram demonstrates the size and configuration of the heart chambers, the shape and function of the valves, and the thickness and contractility of the heart's muscular walls. Echocardiography can also show if a septal defect or other structural abnormality is present. Use of color-flow Doppler technology (described later in this chapter) enables detection of even tiny shunts and minor degrees of valvular incompetence.

A cooperative child is necessary for the procedure. If the child is uncooperative, some type of sedation may be needed.

After a diagnosis has been made by echocardiograph, it may then be confirmed with catheterization and angiocardiography. Echocardiography and Doppler ultrasound studies (discussed later in this chapter) are superior to cardiac catheterization and angiography for assessing complete or partial atrioventricular canal (see Chapter 15) and give a good indication of whether the condition is amenable to surgery. Echocardiography and Doppler ultrasound studies are also accurate enough to be the sole diagnostic method in other conditions.

Fetal Echocardiography

In 1980 cardiologists first used ultrasound to identify normal fetal cardiac anatomy. Today accurate diagnosis of fetal cardiac malformations can be made as early as 14 weeks' gestation. By 19 weeks, almost all of the cardiac connections are visible.

Because maternal diabetes increases the risk of congenital heart disease twofold to threefold, cardiologists now routinely perform fetal echocardiography on pregnant diabetic mothers at 19 weeks' gestation. In pregnant patients with insulin-dependent diabetes, the risk of fetal cardiac malformation is high.

Doppler Studies

The Doppler technique employs a transducer to pulse a beam of sound waves toward an object. If the object is moving toward the transducer, the frequency of the reflected sound waves is higher than the frequency of the original sound waves; if the object is moving away, the reflected frequency is lower. This phenomenon is called the **Doppler effect.** In the case of flowing blood, for example, blood moving toward the transducer might be shown in red on a phosphor screen, whereas blood moving away would be shown in blue.

This technique is very useful for assessing the pressure gradient across a valve; that is, the difference in pressure above and below the valve. The gradient is valuable for evaluating the seriousness of flow obstruction by a stenotic valve or other obstructions; a normal valve has no gradient across it. In addition, coarctation of the aorta, aortic insufficiency, and patent ductus arteriosus have characteristic Doppler waveforms.

Cardiac Catheterization and Angiocardiography

Cardiac catheterization and angiocardiography require the insertion of a long tube into the heart through a peripheral blood vessel and the injection of a radiopaque dye. Even when the type of congenital heart disease has been defined by two-dimensional echocardiography and color-flow Doppler studies, catheterization can be important for assessing pulmonary artery size, pulmonary artery pressure, and pulmonary vascular resistance. Catheterization may also be necessary for reliable quantitation of shunts and valvular gradients. Knowledge of pulmonary vascular resistance is very important when the surgeon is contemplating certain corrective procedures.

The Fontan operation (see Chapter 15), for example, will not be successful in a child with high pulmonary vascular resistance.

Catheterization can diagnose all types of congenital heart defects. It is particularly valuable for lesions difficult to detect with echo-Doppler studies, such as vascular rings and total anomalous pulmonary venous connection. If intracardiac surgery is contemplated, an angiogram can indicate whether the coronary arteries might be in the way of the planned incision.

In recent years, catheterization and angiocardiography have been prerequisites for fewer and fewer cases. In most newborns who are blue or who are in heart failure, Doppler and echocardiography may be sufficient to determine what type of congenital heart disease is present. Echo-Doppler studies in such infants are the principal tests helping the clinician to plan for surgical intervention, if necessary.

BIBLIOGRAPHY

Bernstein D: The cardiovascular system. In Behrman RE, Kliegman RM, Jenson HB, editors: **Nelson textbook of pediatrics,** ed 16, Philadelphia, 2000, WB Saunders.

Falkner B, Sadowski RH: Hypertension in children and adolescents. In Moller JH, Hoffman JI, editors: **Pediatric cardiovascular medicine,** Philadelphia, 2000, Churchill Livingston.

The fetus and neonatal infant, non-infectious disorders. In Behrman RE, Kliegman RM, Jenson HB, editors: **Nelson textbook of pediatrics,** ed 16, Philadelphia, 2000, WB Saunders.

Friedman WF, Silverman N: Congenital heart disease in infancy and childhood. In Braunwald E, Zipes DP, Libby P, editors: **Heart disease,** ed 6, Philadelphia, 2001, WB Saunders.

Johnson MC, Strauss AW: Genetic control in pediatric cardiovascular medicine. In Moller JH, Hoffman JI, editors: **Pediatric cardiovascular medicine,** Philadelphia, 2000, Churchill Livingston.

Lehrer S: **Understanding lung sounds,** ed 3, Philadelphia, 2001, WB Saunders.

Liebman J: Diagnosis and management of heart murmurs in children, **Pediatr Rev** 3:312-329, 1982.

McKusick VA: **Cardiovascular sound in health and disease,** Baltimore, 1958, Williams & Wilkins.

Moller JH: Clinical history and physical examination. In Moller JH, Hoffman JI, editors: **Pediatric cardiovascular medicine,** Philadelphia, 2000, Churchill Livingston.

Nadas AS, Fyler DC: **Pediatric cardiology,** ed 3, Philadelphia, 1972, WB Saunders.

Park MK: **Pediatric cardiology for practitioners,** ed 3, St Louis, 1996, Mosby.

Perloff JK: **Physical examination of the heart and circulation,** ed 3, Philadelphia, 2000, WB Saunders.

Strauss AW: The molecular basis of congenital cardiac disease, **Semin Thorac Cardiovasc Surg Pediatr Card Surg Annu** 1:179-188, 1998.

Teitel D, Heymann MA, Liebman J: The heart. In Klaus M, Fanaroff A, editors: **Care of the high risk neonate,** ed 3, Philadelphia, 1986, WB Saunders.

Vetter V: Arrhythmias. In Moller JH, Hoffman JI, editors: **Pediatric cardiovascular medicine,** Philadelphia, 2000, Churchill Livingston.

Vyse TJ: Sphygmomanometer bladder length and measurement of blood pressure in children, **Lancet** 1:561-562, 1987.

Chapter 4

Phonocardiography and the Recording of External Pulses

Although phonocardiography and external pulse recording are no longer commonly used in the diagnosis of heart disease, an understanding of the principles underlying these techniques helps to clarify the physiology of the action of the heart and sound generation.

PHONOCARDIOGRAPHY

Phonocardiography is the graphic recording of the sounds of the heart. In addition to serving as a check on the accuracy of heart sounds as heard, the phonocardiogram is an excellent teaching tool. There are two principal methods of phonocardiography, oscillographic and spectral.

In the **oscillographic method,** which is in general use, the time scale is represented on the horizontal axis and sound intensity on the vertical axis. Counting the number of peaks or oscillations per second provides an estimate of the frequency of a sound.

The **spectral method** employs a device known as a sound spectrograph, which displays the time scale on the horizontal axis and the sound frequency on the vertical axis. Sound intensity is represented by the darkness of the tracing. The spectral sound recording can convey considerably more information than an oscillographic recording. In fact, in spectral recording of speech individual words can be discerned, which is not possible with oscillographic recordings. Spectral recordings of heart sounds are especially well suited to the demonstration of the musical quality of a murmur (Figures 4-1 and 4-2).

Standard oscillographic phonocardiograph machines contain additional channels for simultaneous recording of the electrocardiogram, carotid pulse tracing, jugular pulse tracing, and apexcardiogram. These recordings serve as useful references for sound interpretation.

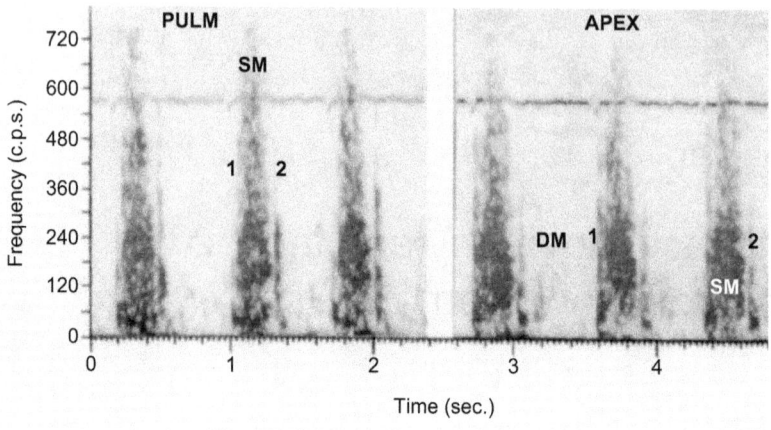

FIGURE 4-1. Sound spectrogram of the systolic murmur **(SM)** of aortic stenosis in a seven-year-old child. Note the irregular texture of the murmur, indicating that it is nonmusical. The apex, as opposed to the pulmonic area **(PULM)**, has an early diastolic murmur **(DM)**, probably of mitral origin, since it begins just after the second heart sound **(2)**. **1,** First heart sound; **c.p.s.,** cycles per second. (From McKusick VA: **Cardiovascular sound in health and disease,** Baltimore, 1958, Williams & Wilkins.)

ELECTROCARDIOGRAPHY

The electrocardiogram (ECG) is the most commonly used reference tracing in the study of heart sounds (see Chapter 1). Because the QRS complex immediately precedes mechanical contraction of the heart, the ECG serves as a reliable guide to ventricular systole and associated heart sounds (Figure 4-3).

CAROTID PULSE TRACING

In Figure 4-4 a normal carotid pulse tracing (CPT) is shown in relationship to the ECG and the phonocardiogram. The curve reflects the volume changes occurring in a segment of the carotid artery with each heartbeat. These changes bear a striking resemblance to pressure changes within the vessel. Because of its relationship to the heart and great vessels, the carotid pulse closely mirrors the aortic pressure pulse.

The CPT consists of a series of deflections, illustrated in Figure 4-4.

With aortic ejection, the carotid pulse tracing rises sharply, reaching its first peak, the percussion wave or **P wave,** when ejection is maximal.

A plateau or secondary wave, the tidal wave or **T wave,** occurs late in systole. Current physiologic studies indicate that the T wave is primarily a reflected pulse wave returning from the periphery.

The **dicrotic notch** (D) represents aortic closure. It is seen 0.02 to 0.05 second later because of the time required for the pulse to travel to the neck.

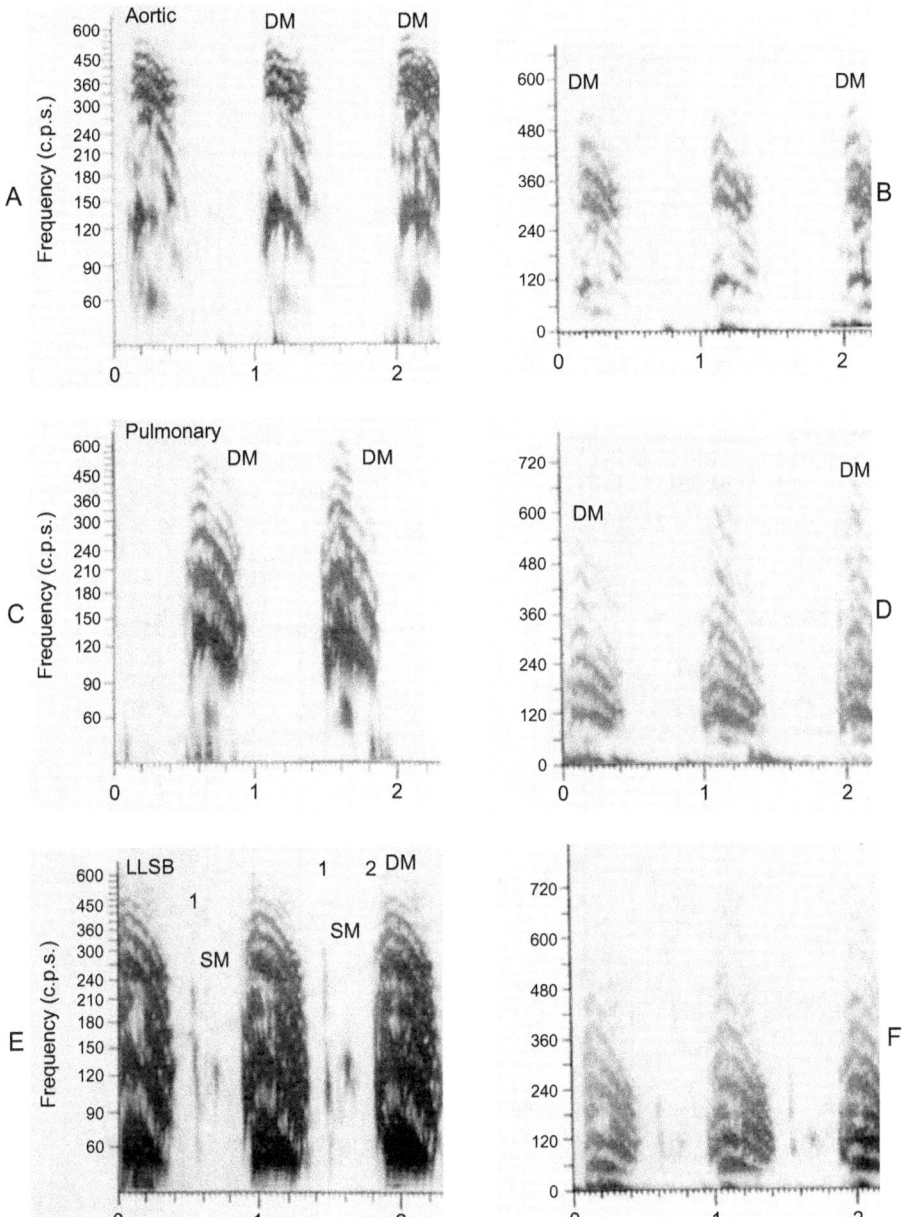

FIGURE 4-2. The diastolic murmur **(DM)** caused by a retroverted (backward-turned) aortic cusp. The frequency is displayed logarithmically **(left)** and linearly **(right).** The record was made in the aortic **(A** and **B)**, pulmonary **(C** and **D)**, and lower left sternal border **(LLSB)** areas **(E** and **F).** Note the semihorizontal bands, the harmonics, indicating the musical quality of the murmur. **1,** First heart sound; **2,** second heart sound; **c.p.s.,** cycles per second; **SM,** systolic murmur. (From McKusick VA: **Cardiovascular sound in health and disease,** Baltimore, 1958, Williams & Wilkins.)

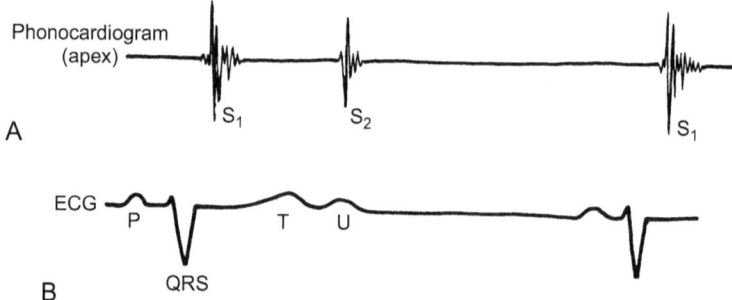

FIGURE 4-3. The relationship between a phonocardiogram and an electrocardiogram. Note that the QRS complex precedes mechanical contraction of the heart (the interval between S_1 and S_2). Note also that the T wave precedes S_2, while the U wave follows it. The U wave is a small wave of low voltage that follows the T wave. It normally has the same polarity as the T wave—that is, if the T wave is upright, the U wave is upright. The U wave is most visible in the midprecordial leads, V_3 to V_4, and is accentuated in patients with low serum potassium and an abnormally slow heart rate.

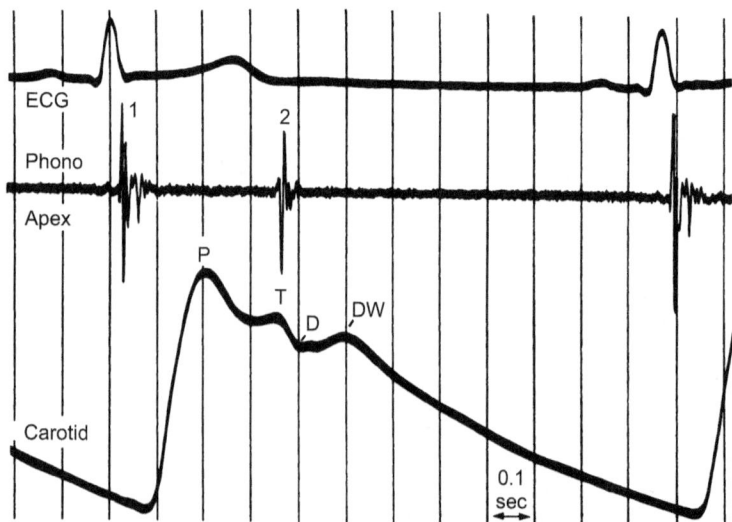

FIGURE 4-4. Normal carotid pulse, showing percussion wave **(P)**, tidal wave **(T)**, dicrotic notch **(D)** and dicrotic wave **(DW)**. **1,** First heart sound; **2,** second heart sound. (From Tavel ME: **Clinical phonocardiography and external pulse recording,** ed 4, Chicago, 1985, Year

This travel time is least in patients with high systolic pressure. The dicrotic notch is a useful reference point because the aortic component of the second heart sound (A_2) always precedes it. The pulmonary component of the second sound (P_2) follows the dicrotic notch in normal patients and varies with respiration.

The **dicrotic wave** (DW) appears early in diastole. It is thought to represent the pulse as it is reflected from the distal arterial tree.

Ejection sounds may be identified on the phonocardiogram by using the CPT. These sounds are high-frequency transients, sometimes called **ejection clicks.** They follow the first heart sound very closely and correspond with the initial rapid ascent of the carotid pulse.

JUGULAR PULSE TRACING

The jugular pulse tracing (JPT) reflects changes in the right atrium. Jugular pulse and right atrial tracings are quite similar, despite the fact that the former reflects volume fluctuations in the jugular vein, whereas the latter indicates pressure changes in the right atrium.

The normal JPT is composed of the series of waves illustrated in Figure 4-5.

The initial **A wave** is caused by right atrial contraction. It is normally the highest point in the cycle, and its summit may coincide with the fourth heart sound or occur up to 0.02 second after.

The **C wave,** which follows, is now thought to be caused chiefly by tricuspid closure. In the past, it was thought that the C wave was solely the result of carotid arterial interference.

The **X descent** is caused by atrial relaxation and perhaps, to a lesser degree, by motion of the right ventricle or valve ring. The X descent begins with the down slope of the A wave, is interrupted by the C wave, and then continues to the **X trough,** which occurs late in systole, 0.09 second before the second heart sound. Some investigators break the X descent into two phases, the X descent preceding the C wave and the X_1 descent thereafter.

The **V wave** is caused by the filling of the right atrium while the tricuspid valves are closed. It begins shortly before the second heart sound and reaches its peak 0.06 to 0.08 second after pulmonic valve closure. (These time values reflect an adolescent or adult heart rate, and would be less in small children.)

The **Y descent** commences with the opening of the tricuspid valve and reaches the Y trough around the end of the early diastolic right atrial emptying. The Y trough is seen 0.20 second after pulmonary closure.

An **H wave,** which is present only in a long cycle, indicates the end of right ventricular filling.

APEXCARDIOGRAPHY

The apexcardiogram (ACG) graphically demonstrates the low-frequency vibrations of the chest wall over the point of maximal impulse. These vibrations are of large amplitude and, to some extent, can be appreciated with the fingertips. Because of the position of the heart and the placement of the pickup device, it is thought that the ACG normally reflects events taking place predominantly or solely in the left ventricle. The ACG is of value in detecting and identifying the mitral opening snap and the third and fourth heart sounds. In contrast to the JPT and the CPT, the ACG provides an instantaneous, undelayed representation of the underlying cardiovascular events.

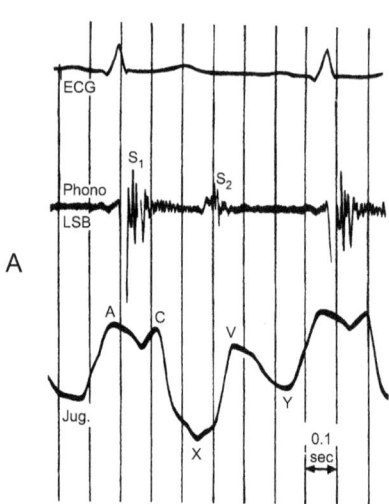

FIGURE 4-5. Examples of normal jugular pulse tracings. **A,** The A wave is the highest deflection, and the **X** trough represents the lowest point on the tracing. **B,** The heart rate is sufficiently slow to allow for the appearance of an H wave in late diastole. **LSB,** Left sternal border. (From Tavel ME: **Clinical phonocardiography and external pulse recording,** ed 4, Chicago, 1985, Year Book.)

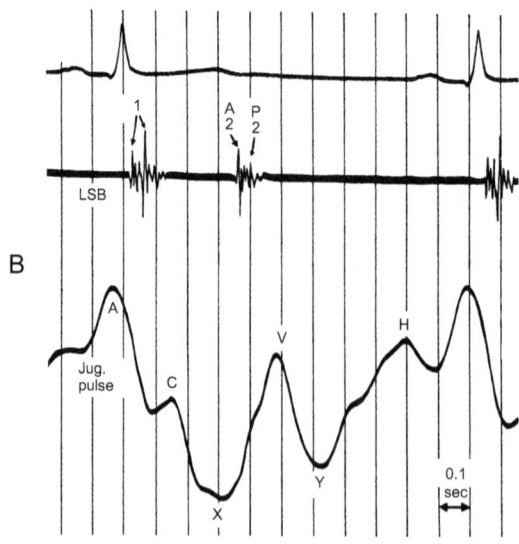

The normal ACG consists of the following deflections (Figure 4-6).

The **A wave** is a small peak that occurs at the instant of left atrial contraction. The peak of the A wave coincides with the fourth heart sound.

The **isovolumic contraction interval** immediately follows the C point and corresponds with the initial part of the first heart sound.

The **E point** indicates the onset of blood ejection from the ventricle into the aorta and coincides with the third component of the first heart sound. The E point is followed by a rapid fall, occurring during the initial rapid ejection phase of left ventricular systole. Just after aortic closure, the curve descends sharply, signifying the end of isovolumic relaxation.

The **O point** is a trough marking the end of the downward fall of the tracing, occurring at approximately the time of mitral valve opening.

After the O point, the curve rises steeply and is labeled the **rapid-filling (RF) wave,** which corresponds with the third heart sound. The RF wave

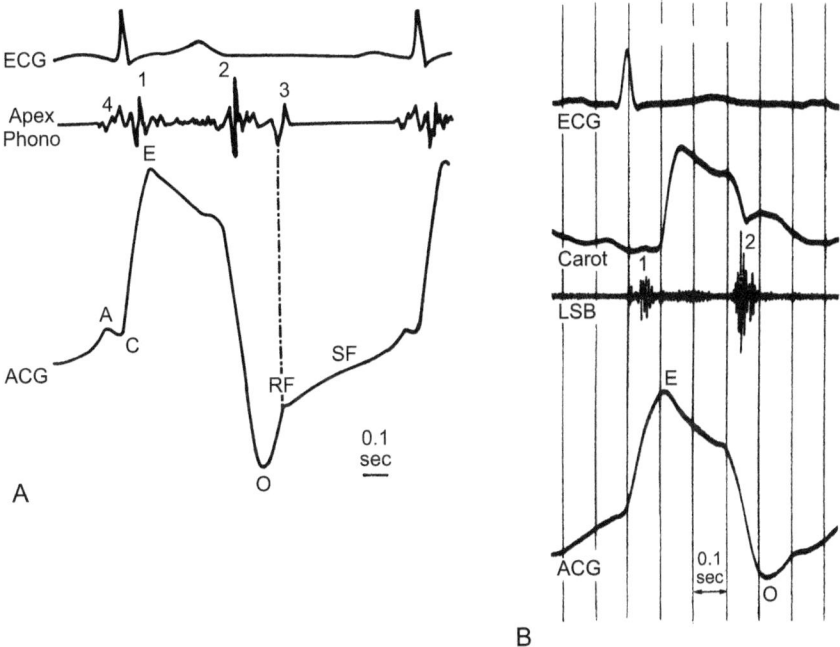

FIGURE 4-6. Examples of apexcardiograms (ACGs) in normal individuals. A, Typical ACG from a normal youth with audible physiologic third heart sound. The rapid-filling **(RF)** wave is peaked and halts abruptly with a subsequent small retraction, and the third heart sound coincides with this peak. The A wave of the ACG represents ventricular motion in response to atrial contraction. B, Normal ACG together with carotid pulse and sounds. In this instance, the ACG shows no clearly discernible A wave. The **E** point of the ACG coincides with the beginning upstroke of the carotid pulse. **C,** Beginning of left-ventricular contraction; **E,** beginning of left-ventricular ejection; **LSB,** left sternal border; **O,** mitral opening; **SF,** slow-filling wave. (From Tavel ME: **Clinical phonocardiography and external pulse recording,** ed 4, Chicago, 1985, Year Book.)

generally reaches a sharp point, sometimes called the **F point.**

Thereafter the tracing continues upward less steeply, a segment referred to as the **slow-filling (SF) wave.** The gentle incline is associated with the slower, passive ventricular filling.

BIBLIOGRAPHY

Castellanos A, Interian A Jr, Myerburg RJ: The resting electrocardiogram. In Fuster V, Alexander RW, O'Rourke RA, editors: **Hurst's the heart,** New York, 2001, McGraw Hill.

Friedman WF, Silverman N: Congenital heart disease in infancy and childhood. In Braunwald E, Zipes DP, Libby P, editors: **Heart disease,** ed 6, Philadelphia, 2001, WB Saunders.

Johnson RJ, Swartz MH: **A simplified approach to electrocardiography,** Philadelphia, 1986, WB Saunders.

Liebman J, Plonsey R: Basic principles for understanding electrocardiography, **Pediatrician** 2:251, 1973.

McKusick VA: **Cardiovascular sound in health and disease,** Baltimore, 1958, Williams & Wilkins.

Tavel ME: **Clinical phonocardiography and external pulse recording,** ed 4, Chicago, 1985, Year Book.

Tilkian AG, Conover MB: **Understanding heart sounds and murmurs,** ed 3, Philadelphia, 2001, WB Saunders.

Chapter 5

Auscultation Areas

The choice of where and how to listen for heart sounds has a significant impact on how successful the examination will be. In this chapter, the four traditional areas of auscultation, as well as more recently defined areas, are described. Some suggestions for choosing among them are presented at the end of the chapter.

TRADITIONAL AREAS TO AUSCULTATE

In the nineteenth century, when physicians first developed the methods of cardiac auscultation, four cardinal areas were designated. Although modern studies performed with phonocardiography and cardiac catheterization have shown that these traditional areas of auscultation are much too limited, they nonetheless serve as good points of reference and are frequently alluded to. The traditional areas of auscultation include the following (Figure 5-1):

1. Aortic area: The aortic area is located at the second right intercostal space at the sternal margin.
2. Pulmonic area: The pulmonic area is found at the second left intercostal space at the sternal margin.
3. Tricuspid area: The tricuspid area is at the fourth and fifth intercostal spaces along the lower left sternal border (LLSB).
4. Mitral area: The mitral area is at the cardiac apex (in a normal heart, at the fifth intercostal space at the midclavicular line).

The location of these four areas in relation to the heart valves and the rib cage is shown in Figure 5-2.

REVISED AREAS TO AUSCULTATE

Modern studies of heart sounds have demonstrated that the four traditional areas are inadequate and that better results can be obtained if six areas of the anterior chest wall are auscultated. Auscultation of three additional areas over the back may also yield useful information. The revised auscultatory areas include the left and right ventricular areas, the left and right atrial areas, the aortic area, and the pulmonary area. In children, it is especially important to broaden the traditional areas, because heart valves and chambers may be in unusual locations in the presence of congenital heart malformations.

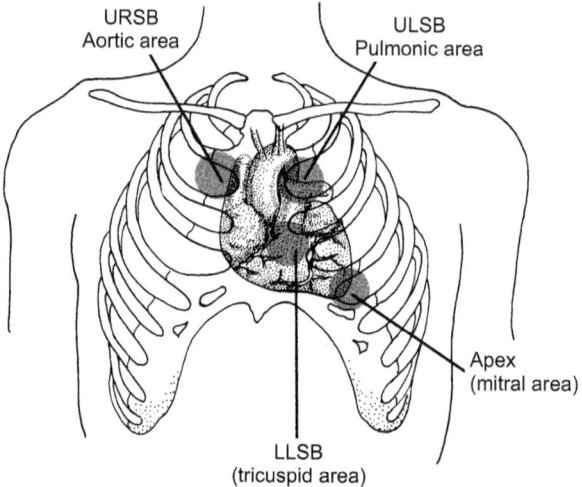

FIGURE 5-1. The traditional areas of auscultation. **LLSB,** Lower left sternal border; **URSB,** upper right sternal border; **ULSB,** upper left sternal border.

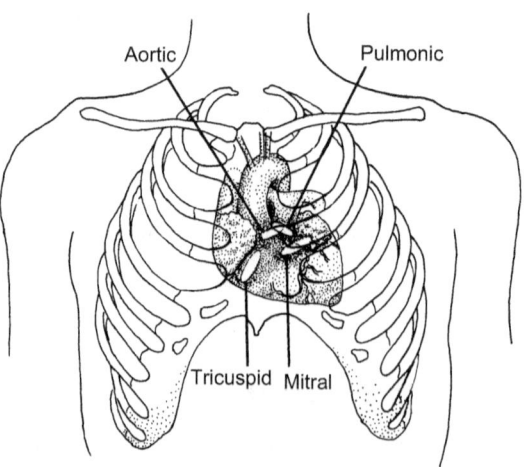

FIGURE 5-2. The location of the heart valves with reference to the rib cage.

Left Ventricular Area

The left ventricular area (Figure 5-3) is centered around the apex of the heart. It extends laterally to the anterior axillary line. When the left ventricle is enlarged, the left ventricular area may be extended medially, to the sternal edge, and also laterally. When the right ventricle is enlarged, the left ventricular auscultation area is displaced to the left.

The following heart sounds are best heard in the left ventricular area:

1. Mitral insufficiency murmur
2. Summation gallops
3. Subaortic stenosis murmur
4. Aortic insufficiency murmur
5. Aortic ejection click in aortic stenosis
6. Click and late systolic murmur in mitral valve prolapse
7. Mitral stenosis murmur: The murmur of organic mitral stenosis is very rare in children; the murmur of relative mitral stenosis, associated with large left-to-right shunts, is more common.

Right Ventricular Area

The right ventricular area (Figure 5-4) encompasses the lower part of the sternum and the third and fourth intercostal spaces on both sides of the sternum. In patients with severe right ventricular enlargement, the right ventricular area may extend to the apical impulse because the apex is then formed by the right ventricle. The following heart sounds are best heard in

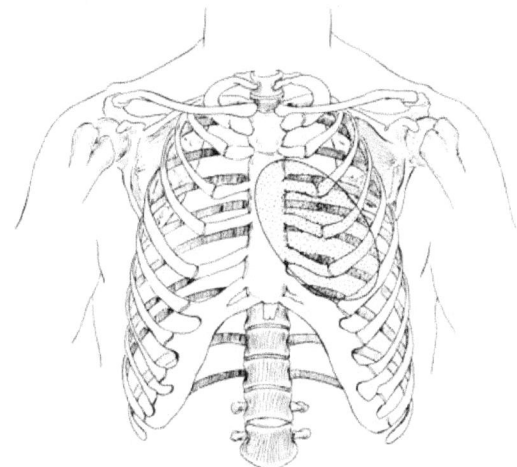

FIGURE 5-3. The left ventricular area.

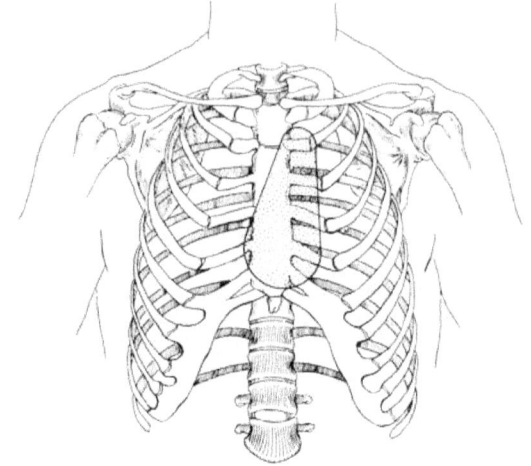

FIGURE 5-4. The right ventricular area.

the right ventricular area:

1. Tricuspid insufficiency murmur
2. Summation gallop
3. Pulmonary insufficiency murmur
4. Ventricular septal defect murmur
5. Aortic insufficiency murmur, especially when the child is sitting
6. Tricuspid stenosis murmur: The murmur of organic tricuspid stenosis is very rare in children, but the murmur of relative tricuspid stenosis is heard in cases of large atrial septal defect and is diagnostic of a large left-to-right shunt.

Left Atrial Area

Murmurs associated with the left atrium (for example, mitral stenosis and mitral insufficiency) are best heard at the apex (Figure 5-5).

Right Atrial Area

The right atrial area extends 1 to 2 cm to the right of the sternum in the fourth and fifth intercostal spaces (Figure 5-6). When the atrium is markedly enlarged, the area reaches to and beyond the right midclavicular line. The murmur of tricuspid insufficiency is best appreciated here.

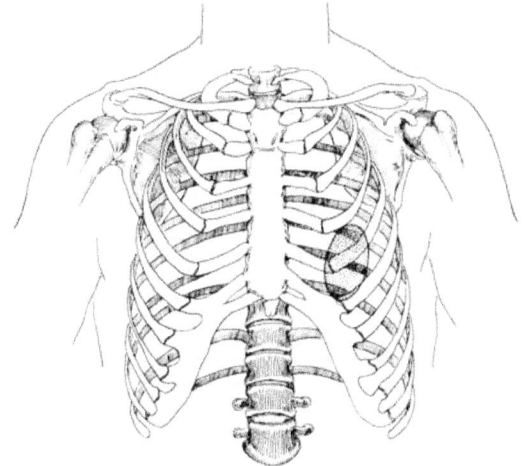

FIGURE 5-5. The left atrial area.

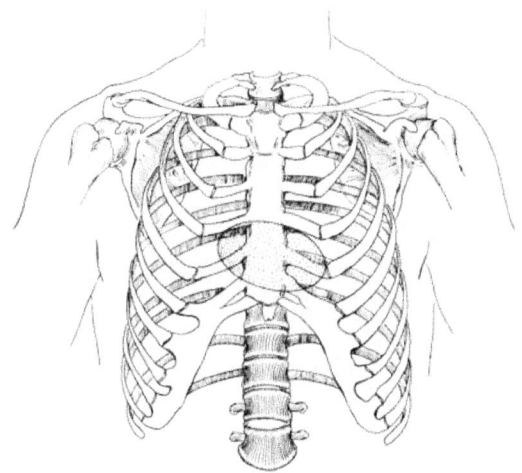

FIGURE 5-6. The right atrial area.

Aortic Area

The aortic area corresponds to the region of the aortic root and part of the ascending aorta (Figure 5-7). It begins at the third left intercostal space and extends across the manubrium to the first, second, and third right intercostal spaces. The aortic area includes the suprasternal notch and the head of the

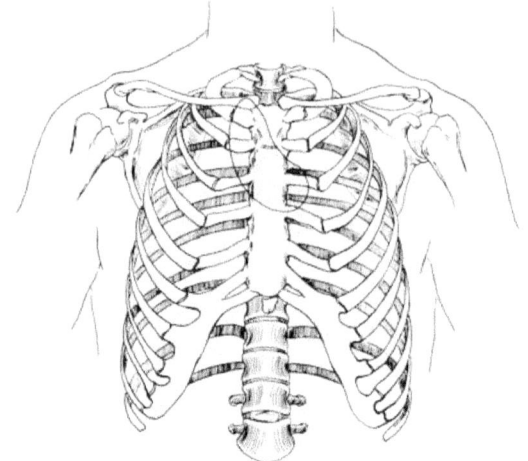

FIGURE 5-7. The aortic area.

right clavicle. The following heart sounds are best heard in the aortic area:

1. Aortic stenosis murmur
2. Aortic insufficiency murmur
3. Sounds caused by increased aortic flow or dilatation of the ascending aorta
4. Sounds produced by abnormalities of the carotid and subclavian arteries
5. The aortic component of the second heart sound (A_2): Aortic murmurs are louder to the right of the sternum if the ascending aorta is dilated. They are louder to the left of the sternum if there is little or no dilatation.

Pulmonary Area

The pulmonary area is an expansion of the traditional area, encompassing the second and third left intercostal spaces close to the sternum (Figure 5-8). The following sounds are best appreciated over the pulmonary area:

1. Pulmonic stenosis murmur
2. Pulmonary insufficiency murmur
3. Murmurs caused by increased flow or dilatation of the pulmonary artery, such as the murmur of atrial septal defect
4. Murmurs caused by stenosis of the main branches of the pulmonary artery
5. The pulmonary ejection click
6. The pulmonary component of the second heart sound (P_2)

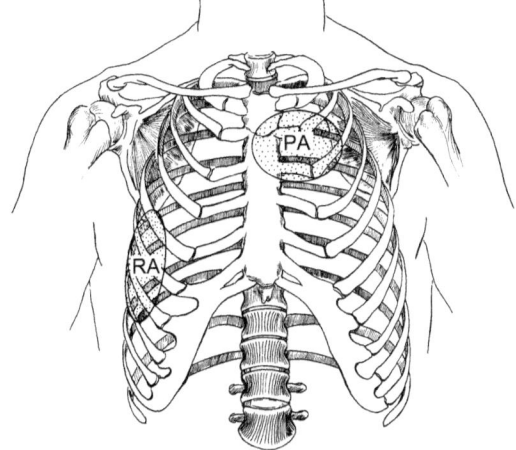

FIGURE 5-8. The pulmonary area. Listening for pulmonary murmurs in the right axilla is often worthwhile, because such murmurs are especially well transmitted to the lung fields. **PA,** Pulmonary area; **RA,** right axilla.

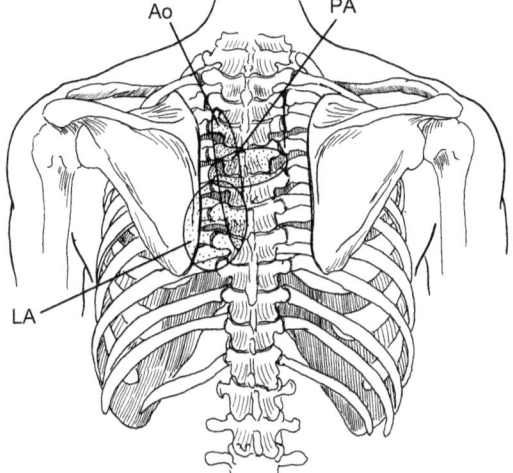

FIGURE 5-9. Areas to auscultate over the back: the left atrial area **(LA),** the aortic area **(Ao),** and the pulmonic area **(PA).** In a child, the only murmurs commonly heard over the back are those generated by shunts, collaterals, and coarctation of the aorta. In practice, many loud murmurs may be audible over the back.

7. Murmur of patent ductus arteriosus

Back and Head

In addition to the six auscultatory areas over the anterior chest, it may be helpful to auscultate the head (arteriovenous fistulas in the brain are audible over the head) and three regions over the back (Figure 5-9). In general, the three listening areas on the back are not as reliable as the six areas over the anterior chest wall. The three back areas include the left atrial area, the aortic area, and the pulmonary area.

1. Left atrial area: The left atrial area overlies the fifth, sixth, seventh, and eighth left posterior intercostal spaces. It is an especially good location to hear the murmur of mitral insufficiency, which sometimes radiates to the back.
2. Aortic area: The aortic area overlies the fourth to eighth thoracic vertebral bodies to the left of the midline. The murmurs of aortic stenosis, aortic insufficiency, and aortic coarctation sometimes may be appreciated here.
3. Pulmonic area: The pulmonic area overlies the fourth and fifth thoracic vertebrae and the corresponding intercostal spaces to the left and right of the spine. The murmurs of pulmonic stenosis, pulmonary insufficiency, and atrial septal defect occasionally radiate to this area.

WHERE SHOULD ONE LISTEN?

Although cardiologists now agree that the traditional listening areas are too limited, they do not universally agree about the revised areas. One successful approach recommended by some clinicians is to listen everywhere, in a systematic fashion, so that no area is missed. The specific area at which an abnormality is heard best is then described. This technique is especially helpful in examining the chest of an infant, because the area to be auscultated is so small. The child should be examined both sitting and lying down, with the bell and the diaphragm of the stethoscope, in every area, including the neck. Radiation to the lateral lung fields may be useful in identifying some murmurs; for example, the murmur of mitral insufficiency is often audible in the axilla, and the murmur of pulmonic stenosis, especially peripheral pulmonic stenosis, radiates especially well to the lung fields.

In auscultating for heart sounds and interpreting results, one should keep in mind that in congenital malformations the vessels, valves, and even the heart itself may be displaced from their usual locations. In rare cases the heart may even be on the right side of the chest (dextrocardia), rather than on the left.

MANEUVERS THAT AID CARDIAC AUSCULTATION

Clinicians may find the following maneuvers useful in auscultating for heart sounds:

1. Exercise: If a murmur is faint or inaudible, it may often be brought out more clearly after exercise.
2. Position: Listening over the apex while the child is lying on the left side (left lateral decubitus position) makes it easier to hear a mitral murmur.
3. End-expiration: Have the child sit up, take a deep breath, exhale, lean

forward, and then hold the breath in end-expiration. This maneuver makes the murmur of aortic insufficiency more audible, especially along the right and left sternal borders at the third intercostal space.

BIBLIOGRAPHY

Liebman J: Diagnosis and management of heart murmurs in children, **Pediatr Rev** 3:321-329, 1982.

Luisada AA: Sounds and pulses as aides to cardiac diagnosis, **Med Clin North Am** 64:3-32, 1980.

McKusick VA: **Cardiovascular sound in health and disease,** Baltimore, 1958, Williams & Wilkins.

Moller JH: Clinical history and physical examination. In Moller JH, Hoffman JI: **Pediatric cardiovascular medicine,** Philadelphia, 2000, Churchill Livingston.

Tilkian AG, Conover MB: **Understanding heart sounds and murmurs,** ed 3, Philadelphia, 2001, WB Saunders.

Chapter 6

The First Heart Sound (S₁)

THE ORIGIN OF S₁

The genesis of the heart sounds, particularly S_1, has long been a controversial subject. In the last few years, sophisticated studies such as high-speed electrocardiograms (ECGs), echocardiograms, phonocardiograms, and carotid and apex pulse tracings have confirmed the origins of the first heart sound. The initial component, M_1, is exactly synchronous with the closure of the mitral valve. Similarly, the second component, T_1, is precisely synchronous with tricuspid valve closure. Both sounds occur with the abrupt cessation of leaflet motion when the cusps have completely closed. The quick deceleration of blood flow and resultant vibration of valves and other structures also contribute to the first heart sound. In complete atrioventricular block (Figure 6-1), in which the mitral valve may close before ventricular contraction, S_1 may be soft or absent, confirming the origins of M_1 and T_1.

THE NATURE OF S₁

The first heart sound is produced when the atrioventricular valves close at the beginning of systole. As Figure 6-2 shows, S_1 has several components: (1) an initial, inaudible low-frequency vibration (M) occurring at the onset of ventricular systole; (2) two intense high-frequency bursts of vibration at the time of atrioventricular valve closure (the first, or mitral, component is called **M_1,** and the second, or tricuspid, component is called **T_1**); and (3) a few low-intensity vibrations. The first sound is low-pitched (duller) and relatively long compared with the second heart sound (S_2) (Figure 6-3).

LISTENING FOR S₁

S_1 is best heard at the apex and can be identified by its relationship to the ECG and carotid upstroke (see Figure 6-2). When the heart is beating very fast, it may be difficult to differentiate the first heart sound from the second. Because the first heart sound always precedes the carotid pulsation, it may be possible to differentiate between them by placing a finger on the carotid pulse while

FIGURE 6-1. Complete atrioventricular block (lead II). (From Guyton AC, Hall JE: **Textbook of medical physiology,** ed 10, Philadelphia, 2000, WB Saunders.)

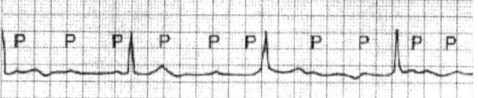

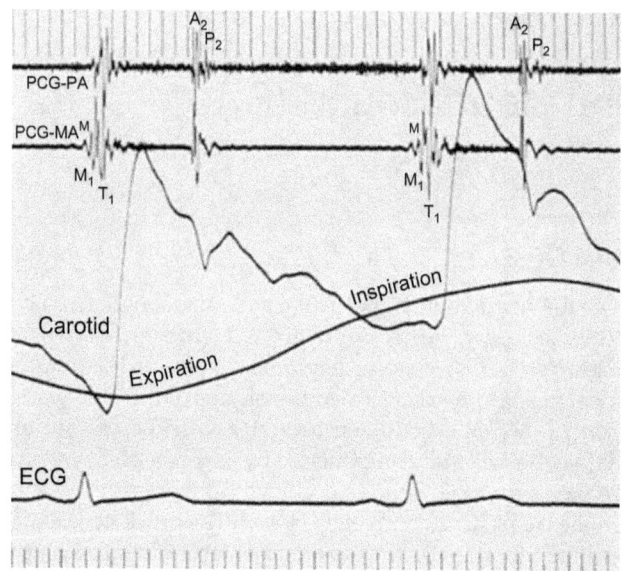

FIGURE 6-2. A normal phonocardiogram showing the first heart sound, best seen at the cardiac apex (PCG-MA). The normal widening of the A_2-P_2 interval with inspiration is demonstrated. **M,** Mitral heart sound; **M_1,** mitral (first heart sound); **PCG-PA,** phonocardiogram—pulmonary area; **T_1,** tricuspid (first heart sound). (From Craige E, Smith D: Heart sounds. In Braunwald E, editor: **Heart disease,** ed 3, Philadelphia, 1988, WB Saunders.)

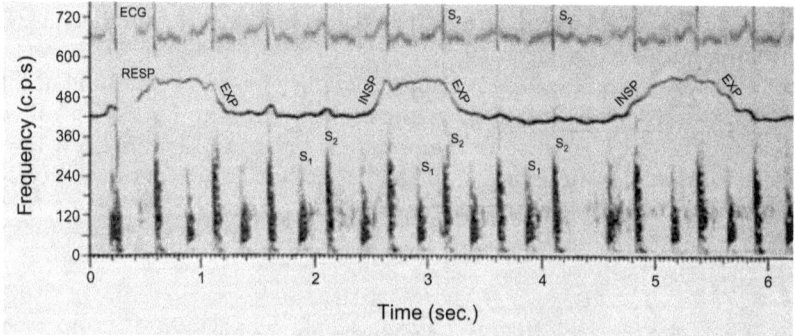

FIGURE 6-3. Pulmonary area in a normal 5-year-old boy. Note the splitting of S_2 late in inspiration and at the beginning of expiration. On the ECG the time of the second heart sound is marked by a vertical line. Note also that S_1 is slightly longer and lower pitched (duller) than S_2. **c.p.s.,** Cycles per second; **EXP,** expiration; **INSP,** inspiration; **RESP,** respiration. (From McKusick VA: **Cardiovascular sound in health and disease,** Baltimore, 1958, Williams & Wilkins.)

listening. S_1 precedes the pulsation, and S_2 comes after.

To hear T_1, the examiner should place the stethoscope over the tricuspid area at the lower left sternal border between the fourth and fifth intercostal spaces. T_1 is much softer than M_1.

SPLITTING OF S₁
Normal Splitting of S₁

Normal splitting of S_1 is often audible in pediatric patients, although it may be difficult to hear, because the gap separating M_1 and T_1 is only 0.02 to 0.03 second. True splitting of S_1 is audible only over the tricuspid area (around the lower left sternal border, usually between the fourth and fifth intercostal spaces at the left sternal edge). What may sound like splitting at the apex is often produced by either (1) a fourth heart sound preceding S_1 or (2) an ejection sound or click, from either the aortic or pulmonic valves, following S_1.

T_1 is softer than M_1 and is always absent at the anterior axillary line. Differentiation of a normally split S_1 from an unsplit S_1 followed by an aortic ejection click depends on this absence of T_1 at the anterior axillary line. If two sounds are audible at the anterior axillary line, the second sound is an aortic ejection click, not the second component of a split first heart sound.

What may be a split S_1, in the absence of a murmur, is likely to be just that, whereas what sounds like a split S_1 in the presence of an ejection murmur is more likely to be a pulmonary or aortic ejection click. Dilatation of either great artery can also give rise to an ejection click in the absence of any valvular abnormality.

Wide Splitting of S₁

Abnormally wide splitting of the first heart sound may occur in the presence of right bundle branch block, ventricular premature contractions, or ventricular tachycardia. In right bundle branch block the wide splitting, as with normal splitting, is best heard over the tricuspid area. In ventricular premature contractions and ventricular tachycardia (Figure 6-4), splitting is heard more easily with the diaphragm of the stethoscope (rather than the bell), because the diaphragm is best for picking up high-pitched vibrations.

INTENSITY OF S₁

The intensity of S_1 may be modified by extracardiac and cardiac factors. The extracardiac factors generally affect both S_1 and S_2, whereas the cardiac factors may influence one sound independent of the other.

Extracardiac Factors Affecting S₁ Intensity

Chest Wall Thickness
The farther a sound has to travel through the chest wall the fainter it is;

FIGURE 6-4. A, Ventricular premature contractions (ectopic beats) are seen alternating with normal beats. The premature contractions have wide, tall QRS complexes.
B, Ventricular tachycardia is characterized by three or more ventricular beats occurring in a run. Both premature ventricular contraction and ventricular tachycardia can cause abnormally wide splitting of the first heart sound. (From Guyton AC, Hall JE: **Textbook of medical physiology,** ed 10, Philadelphia, 2000, WB Saunders.)

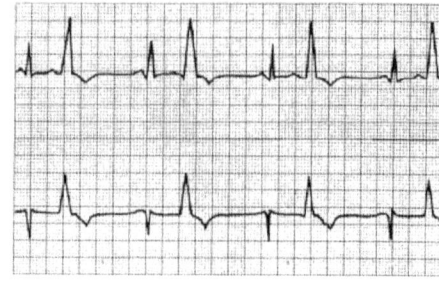

A

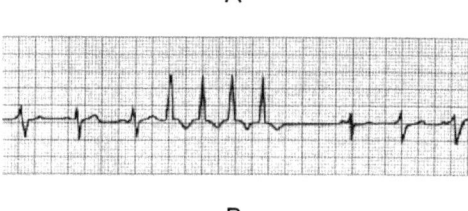

B

therefore, the intensity of S$_1$ is diminished in the presence of conditions, such as obesity or lung disease (e.g., asthma or cystic fibrosis), that increase the anteroposterior diameter of the chest.

Pericardial Fluid
Fluid around the heart may increase the distance that a sound must travel to the chest wall, thereby reducing the intensity of the heart sound. Because sound is better transmitted through fluid than through tissue, however, the greater distance may be offset, and the intensity may not diminish.

Cardiac Factors Affecting S$_1$ Intensity

Position of the Atrioventricular Valve Leaflets
The loudness of S$_1$ is affected by the position of the valve leaflets at the time of ventricular contraction. If the valves are opened wide, they will snap shut with a loud sound. If they are already nearly closed, their complete closing at ventricular contraction generates only a soft sound. An important factor in determining position of the atrioventricular valve leaflets is the P-R interval, which represents the delay between atrial and ventricular contraction. With a prolonged P-R interval (up to 0.25 second—first-degree heart block), S$_1$ is soft, because the mitral valve is almost totally closed when systole begins. When the P-R interval is short, the mitral valve has no time to begin closing before systole. Therefore, the leaflets snap shut quickly and produce a loud S$_1$. S$_1$ is loudest when the P-R interval is at the lower limit of normal.

Forcefulness of Left Ventricular Contraction

The forcefulness of left ventricular contraction can also alter the amplitude of S_1.

Factors producing a **strong contraction** and a **loud S_1** in children include the following:

1. Anemia
2. Thyrotoxicosis
3. Arteriovenous fistula
4. Fever
5. Exercise
6. Anxiety
7. Administration of epinephrine

Factors causing a **weak left ventricular contraction** and a **soft S_1** include the following:

1. Hypothyroidism
2. Cardiomyopathy/myocarditis
3. Shock
4. Left bundle branch block

Pathologic Conditions Affecting S_1 Intensity

Mitral Stenosis

A loud, delayed S_1 is typical of mitral stenosis. In this condition, left atrial pressure is greater than left ventricular end-diastolic pressure, and, as a result, the mitral leaflets are still deep within the ventricle at the onset of left ventricular contraction. In addition, the leaflets are thickened and fibrosed. Both leaflet position and thickening are responsible for the loud S_1 (see Chapter 12). Mitral stenosis is extremely rare in children.

Aortic Insufficiency

In patients with marked aortic insufficiency, S_1 is reduced in amplitude or may even be absent. The reduction may be caused by a prematurely closed mitral valve, a short isovolumic systole, or both.

BEAT-TO-BEAT VARIATIONS OF S_1

A repetitive change in the timing of atrial and ventricular contraction or alteration in the rate of ventricular filling indicates that a beat-to-beat variation of S_1 is occurring (Figure 6-5).

BIBLIOGRAPHY

Braunwald E, Perloff JK: Physical examination of the heart and circulation. In

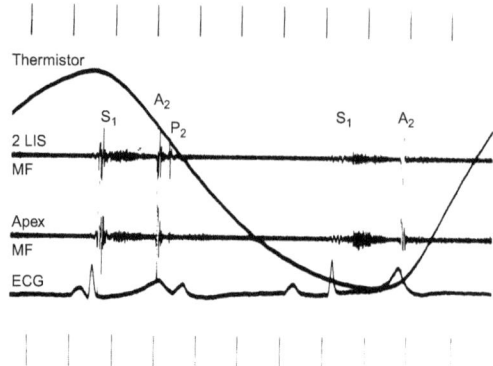

FIGURE 6-5. Beat-to-beat variation of the intensity of the first heart sound (S_1) with varying P-R interval. Note the soft first heart sound when the P-R interval is long **(right)** and compare with the loud first heart sound when the P-R interval is short **(left)**. The thermistor indicates the phase of respiration, with inspiration on the left and expiration on the right. Note the normal splitting of A_2 and P_2 on inspiration. **2LIS,** Second left intercostal space; **MF,** medium frequency. (From Nadas AS, Fyler DC: **Pediatric cardiology,** ed 3, Philadelphia, 1972, WB Saunders. Copyright AS Nadas.)

Braunwald E, Zipes DP, Libby P, editors: **Heart disease,** ed 6, Philadelphia, 2001, WB Saunders.

Friedman WF, Silverman N: Congenital heart disease in infancy and childhood. In Braunwald E, Zipes DP, Libby P, editors: **Heart disease,** ed 6, Philadelphia, 2001, WB Saunders.

Leech G, Brooks N, Green-Wilkinson A et al: Mechanism of influence of PR interval on loudness of first heart sound, **Br Heart J** 43:138-142, 1980.

Levine S, Harvey WP: **Clinical auscultation of the heart,** ed 2, Philadelphia, 1959, WB Saunders.

Luisada AA: Sounds and pulses as aids to cardiac diagnosis, **Med Clin North Am** 64:3-32, 1980.

Luisada AA, MacCanon DM, Kumar S et al: Changing views on the mechanism of the first and second heart sounds, **Am Heart J** 88:503-514, 1974.

McKusick VA: **Cardiovascular sound in health and disease,** Baltimore, 1958, Williams & Wilkins.

Mills PG, Chamusco RF, Moos S et al: Echocardiographic studies of the contribution of the atrioventricular valves to the first heart sound, **Circulation** 54:944-951, 1976.

Nadas AS, Fyler DC: **Pediatric cardiology,** ed 3, Philadelphia, 1972, WB Saunders.

O'Rourke RA, Shaver JA, Silverman ME: The history, physical examination, and cardiac auscultation. In Fuster V, Alexander RW, O'Rourke RA, editors: **Hurst's the heart,** New York, 2001, McGraw Hill.

Ravin A, Craddock LD, Wolf PS et al: **Auscultation of the heart,** ed 3, Chicago, 1977, Year Book.

Talamo RC: Emphysema and alpha-1-antitrypsin deficiency. In Kending EL, Chernick V, editors: **Disorders of the respiratory tract in children,** ed 4, Philadelphia, 1983, WB Saunders.

Tavel ME: **Clinical phonocardiography and external pulse recording,** ed 4, Chicago, 1985, Year Book.

Tilkian AG, Conover MB: **Understanding heart sounds and murmurs,** ed 3, Philadelphia, 2001, WB Saunders.

Chapter 7

The Second Heart Sound (S₂)

Careful evaluation of the second heart sound provides a valuable and simple test of cardiac function. Once the two components, A_2 and P_2, have been identified, their intensities and degree of separation provide vital clues to the presence of many diseases. In addition, respiratory variations in S_2 are particularly important in the diagnosis of heart disease in children.

THE ORIGIN OF S₂

Modern studies have demonstrated that the semilunar valves close silently. The vibrations of the closed valves are the source of S_2. When shut, the valves form stretched, circular membranes that are thin, compliant, and tense. These membranes are set into motion by the surrounding blood just after valve closure, and they vibrate like a diaphragm, generating pressure changes that are audible as sound.

Figure 7-1 shows the two components of S_2 in relation to other events of the cardiac cycle. Note that A_2 (aortic valve closure) is coincident with the end of the left ventricular ejection period and that P_2 (pulmonic valve closure) is coincident with the end of the right ventricular ejection period. P_2 normally occurs after A_2, because right ventricular ejection terminates after left ventricular ejection.

THE NATURE OF S₂

As discussed in Chapter 6, S_2 is sharper in quality (higher pitched) than S_1. Several factors influence the amplitude of S_2, including the following:

1. **The flexibility of the valve leaflets.** When the valve leaflets are calcified or thickened, the valves produce a diminished S_2.
2. **The diameter of the valve.** Dilatation of the aorta or pulmonary artery increases the valve diameter and augments the amplitude of S_2.
3. **Blood viscosity.** In a person with diminished blood viscosity, such as occurs in anemia, S_2 is increased in amplitude.

FIGURE 7-1. The cardiac cycle, recorded by high-fidelity catheter-tipped micromanometers. The aortic (A$_2$) and pulmonic (P$_2$) closure sounds are coincident with the incisurae (notches) of their respective arterial traces (**AO**, aorta; **PA**, pulmonary artery) and are indicated by the vertical dashed lines. Although the durations of right and left ventricular electromechanical systole are nearly equal, note that the right ventricular (**RV**) systolic ejection period terminates after left ventricular (**LV**) ejection, causing physiologic splitting of S$_2$. (From Shaver JA, O'Toole JD: The second heart sound: newer concepts, **Mod Concepts Cardiovasc Dis** 46:1, 1977. By permission of the American Heart Association, Inc.)

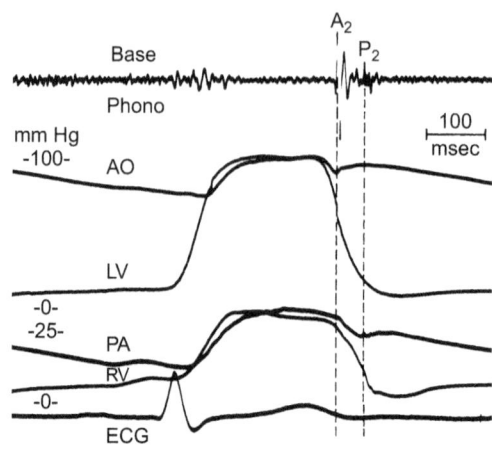

NORMAL (PHYSIOLOGIC) SPLITTING OF S$_2$

During expiration, the aortic and pulmonic valves close at almost the same time, producing a single or closely split S$_2$. During inspiration, the valves close asynchronously, and the aortic valve closes before the pulmonic valve (Figures 7-2 and 7-3), widening the split between A$_2$ and P$_2$ audibly.

Most of the separation results from a delay in pulmonic valve closure related to lower resistance in the pulmonary circulation. During inspiration, intrathoracic pressure is decreased, and the pressure difference between the right atrium and the extrathoracic veins is increased. As a result, blood flow into the right atrium increases and filling of the right ventricle increases. The increased stroke volume of the right ventricle prolongs its systole and retards closure of the pulmonic valve.

Normal inspiratory splitting of S$_2$ is heard in all healthy children, but this splitting is usually absent in newborns and only becomes evident when resistance in the pulmonary circulation falls in the weeks after birth (see Chapter 1).

Listening for the Splitting of S$_2$

Splitting of the second sound is most prominent at the peak or immediately after the peak of inspiration. It can be heard only where both the pulmonary and aortic second sounds are audible; that is, along the high left sternal border at the second to fourth (Figure 7-4). P$_2$ is audible only in this region, whereas A$_2$ is more widely transmitted over the precordium and the lower neck. A$_2$ is also louder than P$_2$.

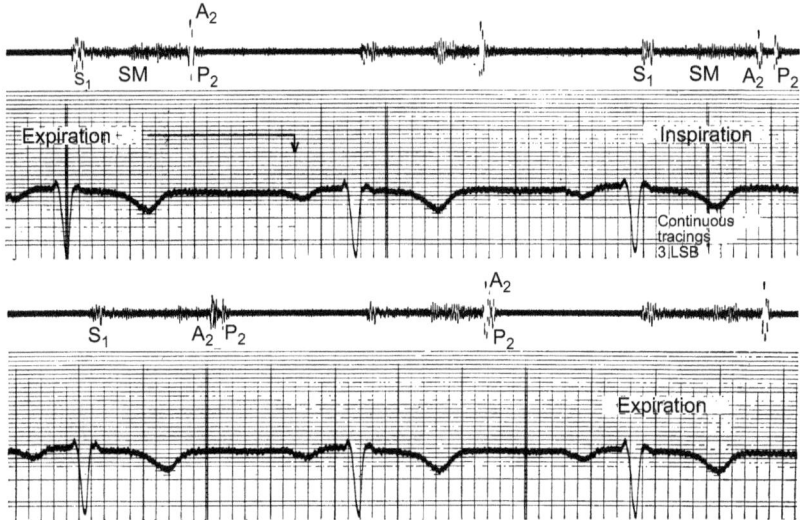

FIGURE 7-2. Normal increase in splitting of second sound with inspiration. **SM,** Systolic murmur. (From Levine SA, Harvey WP: **Clinical auscultation of the heart,** ed 2, Philadelphia, 1959, WB Saunders.)

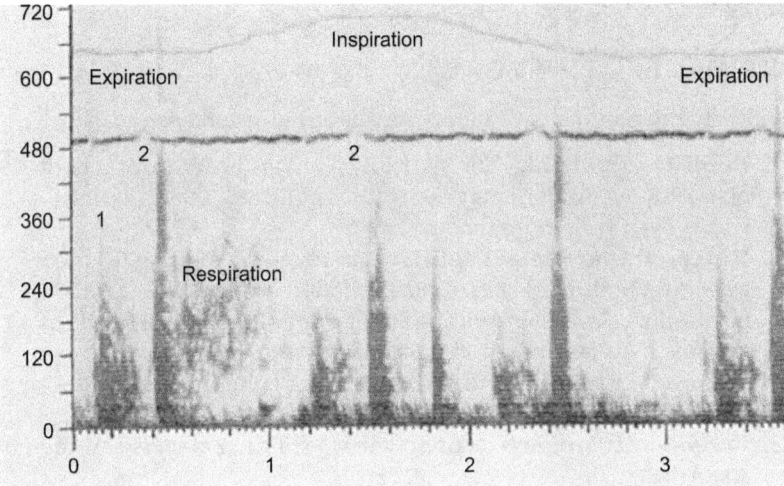

FIGURE 7-3. Sound spectrogram recorded from the pulmonary area in a 13-year-old child. A slight early systolic murmur is present. Note the splitting of S$_2$ on inspiration. Note also that S$_2$ is higher pitched than S$_1$. (From McKusick VA: **Cardiovascular sound in health and disease,** Baltimore, 1958, Williams & Wilkins.)

FIGURE 7-4. The best place to listen for the splitting of S_2.

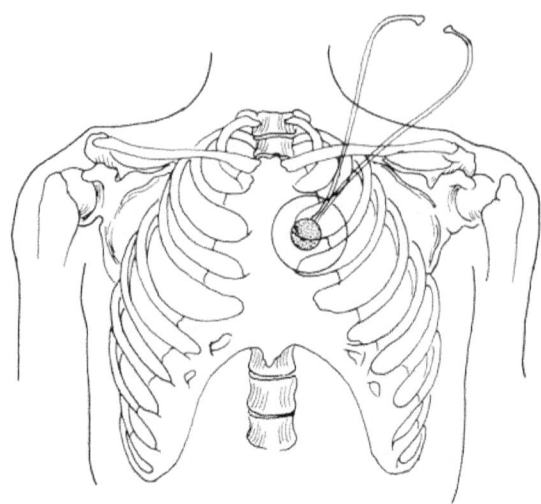

Splitting is best heard with the diaphragm of the stethoscope's chest piece. Any changes in the loudness of the second sound or degree of splitting should be carefully noted. Changes in the quality or pitch of S_2 may also be noted, but these are less important.

ABNORMAL SPLITTING OF S_2

The following variations may signify an abnormal second sound:

1. **Persistent splitting.** The splitting, which is heard during both phases of respiration, may be fixed or nonfixed; that is, it may widen even further on inspiration.
2. **Reversed (paradoxic) splitting.** In reversed splitting, P_2 occurs before A_2. Splitting is heard on expiration and disappears on inspiration. Reversed splitting is very rare. It occurs as the most extreme manifestation of the conditions more commonly causing narrowed splitting. Narrowed splitting is quite frequent and difficult to distinguish from single S_2.
3. **Persistently single S_2.** An S_2 with no splitting at all is considered abnormal.

Persistent Splitting of S_2

When persistent splitting of S_2 is present, the two components, A_2 and P_2, are heard on both inspiration and expiration. Persistent splitting may be a normal finding in a child or adolescent. However, the following variations of persistent splitting may indicate cardiac disease.

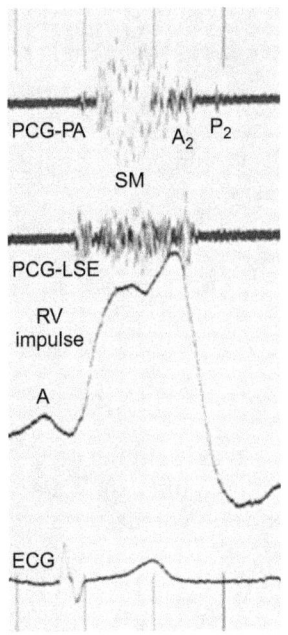

PCG-PA   A₂ P₂

SM

PCG-LSE

RV
impulse

A

ECG

FIGURE 7-5. Wide splitting of S₂ in infundibular pulmonic stenosis. An associated ventricular septal defect is present, with left-to-right shunting. The separation of A_2 and P_2 is 0.08 second, a figure consistent with the systemic pressures encountered in the right ventricle **(RV)**. An ejection murmur occurs in the second left intercostal space **(PA)** from the RV outflow obstruction, whereas at the lower sternal edge **(LSE),** the murmur has a holosystolic configuration, suggesting that the murmur is largely the result of ventricular septal defect. The RV impulse recorded at LSE shows a prominent **a** wave **(A)** and a sustained systolic thrust consistent with right ventricular hypertrophy. **PCG,** Phonocardiogram; **SM,** systolic murmur. (From Craige E, Smith D: Heart sounds. In Braunwald E, editor: **Heart disease,** ed 3, Philadelphia, 1988, WB Saunders.)

Wide Nonfixed Persistent Splitting of S₂ With Respiratory Variation

Wide nonfixed persistent splitting of S₂ may occur for either hemodynamic or electrical reasons.

Hemodynamic Forces

Hemodynamic causes of wide persistent splitting include the following:

1. **Obstruction of right ventricular outflow.** Right ventricular outflow obstruction may be caused by either pulmonic valve stenosis or pulmonary infundibular (outflow tract) stenosis. In both conditions, right ventricular systole is lengthened, and P₂ is delayed and reduced in amplitude. The greater the severity of stenosis, the longer the delay in P₂ and the wider the splitting (Figure 7-5).
2. **Shortening of left ventricular ejection time.** In patients with severe mitral regurgitation, left ventricular ejection time is unusually short. A₂ is therefore early, resulting in an increased splitting of S₂ that widens further on inspiration.
3. **Dilatation of the main pulmonary artery.** For unknown reasons, some children have a dilated pulmonary artery. The resultant increase in volume diminishes the recoil force on the pulmonic valve and delays closure, further lengthening the split between A₂ and P₂.

Electrical Factors

Electrical reasons for wide persistent splitting of S₂ include the following:

1. **Right bundle branch block.** In this condition, excitation and contraction of the right side of the heart are delayed, resulting in delayed closure of the pulmonic valve and P₂. S₂ is split on expiration, and the split increases further on inspiration (Figure 7-6).
2. **Ventricular premature contractions.** Premature contractions originating in the left side of the heart cause wide QRS complexes and persistent splitting of S₂.

Wide Fixed Splitting of S₂

In patients with **atrial septal defect** (Figure 7-7), wide fixed splitting of S₂ occurs, which is not affected by inspiration or expiration (Figure 7-8). Wide fixed splitting of S₂ is a crucial sign in the clinical identification of this defect, and various mechanisms have been proposed to explain it.

Reversed Splitting of S₂

In reversed (paradoxic) splitting of S₂, pulmonic valve closure precedes aortic valve closure, and splitting of S₂ is heard on expiration and disappears on inspiration—the opposite of the normal occurrence (Figure 7-9). Reversed splitting may be caused by either electrical or hemodynamic factors.

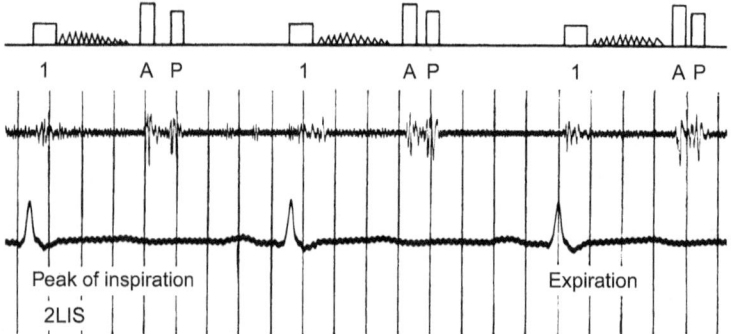

FIGURE 7-6. Increased splitting of second sound in right bundle branch block. The splitting is evident on expiration and becomes more marked on inspiration. The aortic second sound **(A)** precedes the pulmonic second sound **(P).** This patient has a faint systolic murmur, but most of the vibrations, other than the heart sounds, are caused by respiration and muscle noises. **2LIS,** Second left intercostal space. (From Ravin A, Craddock D, Wolf PS et al: **Auscultation of the heart,** ed 3, Chicago, 1977, Year Book.)

Electrical Factors

Any electrical disturbance that alters the normal depolarization of the ventricles can cause reversed splitting of S_2. Among the more common are **left bundle branch block** (which delays left ventricular contraction and

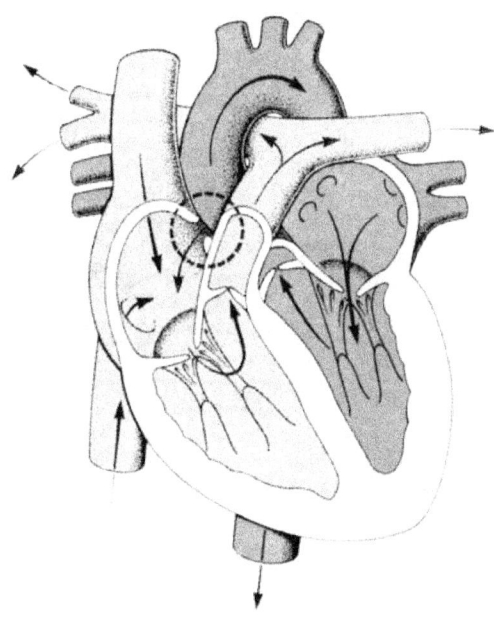

FIGURE 7-7. Atrial septal defect **(circled).** The shunt is from the left atrium to right atrium. (From Foster R, Hunsberger MM, Anderson JT: **Family-centered nursing care of children,** Philadelphia, 1989, WB Saunders.)

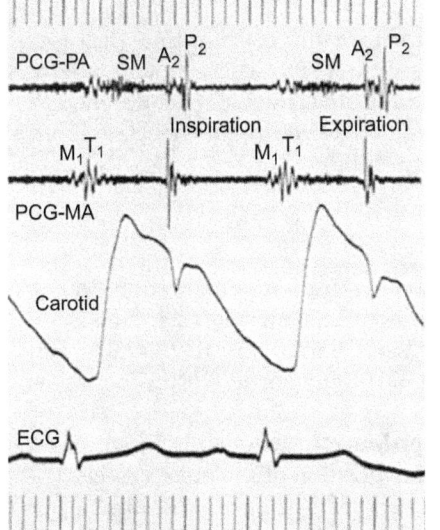

FIGURE 7-8. Atrial septal defect showing a midsystolic murmur **(SM)** and fixed splitting of S_2 in the second left intercostal space **(PCG-PA).** The separation of A_2 and P_2 is 0.06 second in inspiration and expiration. The first heart sound shows a relatively loud tricuspid component **(T₁).** **PCG-MA,** Phonocardiogram—mitral area. (From Craige E, Smith D: Heart sounds. In Braunwald E, editor: **Heart disease,** ed 3, Philadelphia, 1988, WB Saunders.)

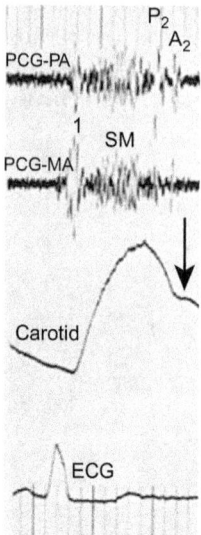

FIGURE 7-9. Aortic stenosis with reversed splitting of S$_2$. A prominent midsystolic murmur is present. A$_2$ is identified by its occurrence immediately prior to the incisura **(arrow)** on the carotid pulse tracing. P$_2$ is seen to fall still earlier by 0.04 second. The carotid upstroke is slow and is shattered by coarse vibrations. **PCG-MA,** Phonocardiogram—mitral area; **PCG-PA,** phonocardiogram—pulmonary area; **SM,** systolic murmur. (From Craige E, Smith D: Heart sounds. In Braunwald E, editor: **Heart disease,** ed 3, Philadelphia, 1988, WB Saunders.)

A$_2$), **ectopic beats, paced beats** (beats induced with an electronic pacemaker), and an abnormal ventricular rhythm originating on the right side of the heart. **Wolff-Parkinson-White syndrome** may cause paradoxic splitting because of early pulmonic valve closure after early excitation of the right ventricle.

Hemodynamic Forces

Mechanical aberrations that prolong left ventricular ejection time delay A$_2$ and can produce narrowed or paradoxic splitting of S$_2$. These include **aortic stenosis** and **left ventricular outflow tract obstruction**. In children with **patent ductus arteriosus,** left ventricular stroke volume and ejection times may be increased, producing paradoxic splitting.

Single S$_2$

In patients with a single S$_2$, no splitting on inspiration or expiration occurs. A single S$_2$, of increased intensity and loudest at the lower left sternal border, is characteristic of **tetralogy of Fallot** (see Chapter 15). In this disorder, pulmonary closure is not audible, and the loud aortic closure sound is transmitted down the descending aorta.

   Pulmonary atresia and severe **pulmonic stenosis** (Figure 7-10) also cause a single S$_2$. In children with transposition of the great vessels, the aorta is in an anterior position, and a single loud S$_2$ may also be audible.

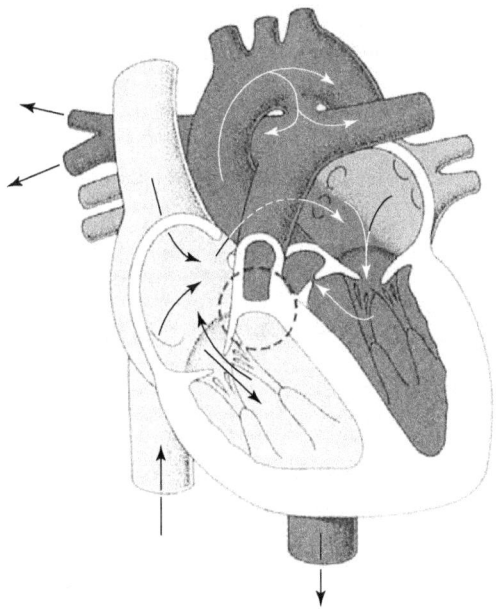

FIGURE 7-10. Pulmonary atresia **(circled area)** with small right ventricle, atrial septal defect (ASD), and patent ductus arteriosus. Abnormal blood flow is from the right chambers through the ASD to the left side of the heart. Blood can reach the lungs only through a patent ductus arteriosus. (From Foster R, Hunsburger MM, Anderson JT: **Family-centered nursing care of children,** Philadelphia, 1989,

AMPLITUDE OF A₂ AND P₂

In addition to the interval between A_2 and P_2, the amplitude of A_2 and P_2 may provide further information about cardiac disease.

Loud P₂

Unless proved otherwise, a loud P_2 is considered to be caused by **pulmonary hypertension** (Figure 7-11). The recognition of pulmonary hypertension is especially important in children with shunts (atrial septal defect, ventricular septal defect, and patent ductus arteriosus), because if hypertension is overlooked, pulmonary vascular changes may become irreversible.

The loud P_2 of pulmonary hypertension is more widely transmitted than P_2 in children without pulmonary hypertension, sometimes to the cardiac apex or to the right of the sternum. The amplitude and transmission of P_2 are only crude indicators of the degree of pulmonary hypertension, and the child with a loud P_2 must be further investigated. If a loud P_2 is associated with a decrescendo diastolic murmur, pulmonary hypertension is usually severe.

Loud A₂

Although an increase in the amplitude of A_2 is more difficult to perceive and quantify than an increase in P_2, a relatively loud A_2 may be detected in patients with **systemic hypertension** or **coarctation of the aorta**. A$_2$ is also loud in either **dextrotransposition** or **levotransposition of the great arteries,** because the aorta is displaced anteriorly. Children with **aortic regurgitation** usually have a loud A$_2$, although it may be soft if the valve is very deformed (Figure 7-12).

Figure 7-13 summarizes the most common changes in the second heart sound.

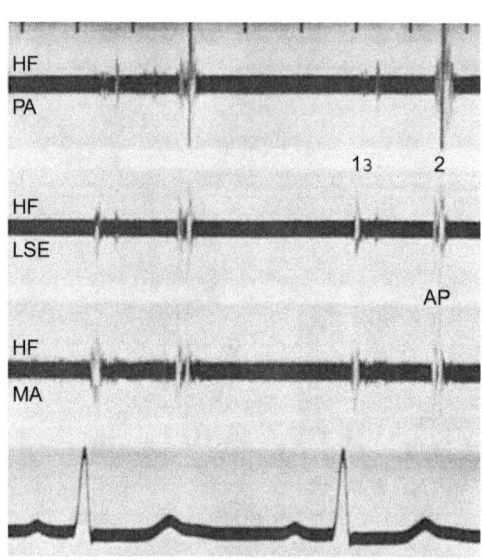

FIGURE 7-11. Pulmonary hypertension. P$_2$ is abnormally loud and dwarfs A$_2$ at the pulmonary area, causing difficulty in auscultation of the two components. The transmission of P$_2$ to the mitral area is abnormal; furthermore, the split can be detected more easily at the mitral area, where the two components are similar in size. **HF,** High frequency; **LSE,** lower sternal edge; **MA,** mitral area; **PA,** pulmonic area. (From Leatham A: **Auscultation of the heart and phonocardiography,** Edinburgh, 1970, Churchill Livingstone.

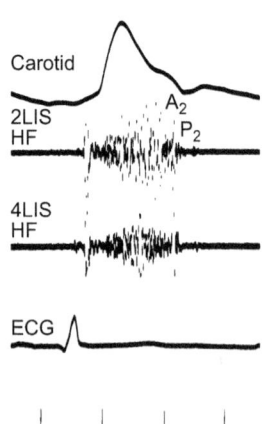

FIGURE 7-12. Phonocardiogram of patient with pulmonic stenosis. The second sound is widely split, with a low-intensity pulmonic component. A diamond-shaped murmur with a late apex is also present. These changes are characteristic of severe stenosis. **HF,** High frequency; **2LIS,** second left intercostal space; **4LIS,** fourth left intercostal space. (From Nadas AS, Fyler DC: **Pediatric cardiology,** ed 3, Philadelphia, 1972, WB Saunders. Copyright AS Nadas.)

EXPIRATION
2LIS

INSPIRATION
2LIS

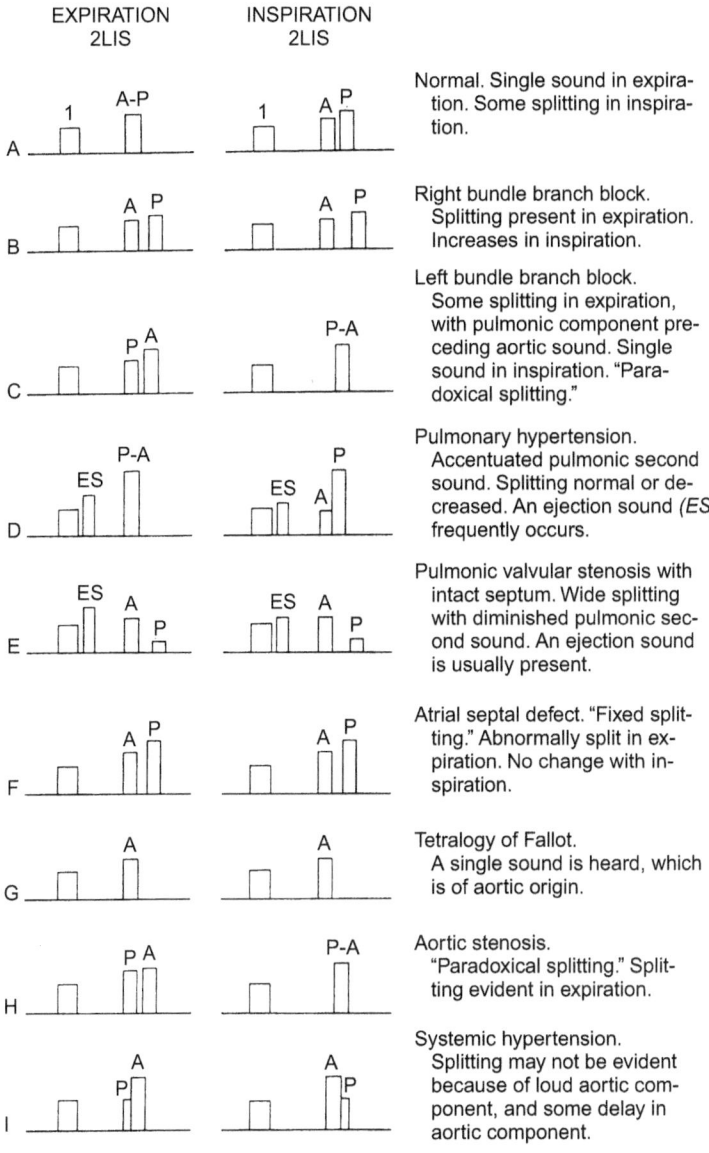

A. Normal. Single sound in expiration. Some splitting in inspiration.

B. Right bundle branch block. Splitting present in expiration. Increases in inspiration.

C. Left bundle branch block. Some splitting in expiration, with pulmonic component preceding aortic sound. Single sound in inspiration. "Paradoxical splitting."

D. Pulmonary hypertension. Accentuated pulmonic second sound. Splitting normal or decreased. An ejection sound *(ES)* frequently occurs.

E. Pulmonic valvular stenosis with intact septum. Wide splitting with diminished pulmonic second sound. An ejection sound is usually present.

F. Atrial septal defect. "Fixed splitting." Abnormally split in expiration. No change with inspiration.

G. Tetralogy of Fallot. A single sound is heard, which is of aortic origin.

H. Aortic stenosis. "Paradoxical splitting." Splitting evident in expiration.

I. Systemic hypertension. Splitting may not be evident because of loud aortic component, and some delay in aortic component.

FIGURE 7-13. Changes in the second sound. **A,** Aortic second sound; **ES,** early ejection sound; **P,** pulmonic second sound; **2LIS,** second left intercostal space. (From Ravin A, Craddock D, Wolf PS et al: **Auscultation of the heart,** ed 3, Chicago, 1977, Year Book.)

BIBLIOGRAPHY

Braunwald E, Perloff JK: Physical examination of the heart and circulation. In Braunwald E, Zipes DP, Libby P, editors: **Heart disease,** ed 6, Philadelphia, 2001, WB Saunders.

Craige E, Harned HS: Phonocardiographic and electrocardiographic studies in normal newborn infants, **Am Heart J** 65:180, 1963.

Levine S, Harvey WP: **Clinical auscultation of the heart,** ed 2, Philadelphia, 1959, WB Saunders.

Liebman J: Diagnosis and management of heart murmurs in children, **Pediatr Rev** 3:321-329, 1982.

Luisada AA: Sounds and pulses as aids to cardiac diagnosis, **Med Clin North Am** 64:3-32, 1980.

McKusick VA: **Cardiovascular sound in health and disease,** Baltimore, 1958, Williams & Wilkins.

O'Rourke RA, Shaver JA, Silverman ME: The history, physical examination, and cardiac auscultation. In Fuster V, Alexander RW, O'Rourke RA, editors: **Hurst's the heart,** New York, 2001, McGraw-Hill.

Ravin A, Craddock LD, Wolf PS et al: **Auscultation of the heart,** ed 3, Chicago, 1977, Year Book.

Sabbah HN, Khaja F, Anbe DT et al: The aortic closure sound in pure aortic insufficiency, **Circulation** 56:859, 1977.

Stein PD, Sabbah HN: Origin of the second heart sound: clinical relevance of new observations, **Am J Cardiol** 41:108-110, 1978.

Tilkian AG, Conover MB: **Understanding heart sounds and murmurs,** ed 3, Philadelphia, 2001, WB Saunders.

Chapter 8

The Third and Fourth Heart Sounds (S$_3$ and S$_4$)

Both the third and fourth heart sounds occur in diastole and are of low frequency. Years ago they were named **gallops,** because they can make the heartbeat sound like a horse running.

IDENTIFYING EXTRA HEART SOUNDS

A technique called **inching** (moving the bell of the stethoscope in small increments) can be used to hear the third and fourth heart sounds and to determine whether an extra sound is systolic or diastolic. This technique depends on the fact that the second heart sound is almost always louder over the aortic area than the first heart sound is. The second heart sound is readily identified by inching the stethoscope from the aortic area to the apex area, because the second sound is louder than the first sound over the aortic area but becomes relatively softer as the bell approaches the apex.

Once the second heart sound has been clearly identified, attention can be focused on the extra sound. If it occurs after the second heart sound or before the first heart sound, the extra sound is diastolic. If the extra sound is heard after the first heart sound but before the second, it is systolic. Even in children with rapid heart rates, the inching technique permits easy, reliable characterization of an extra sound and its identification as either a third or fourth heart sound.

THE THIRD HEART SOUND

The third heart sound is a normal finding in children and young adults. In one study of 1200 schoolchildren 8 to 12 years of age, all had a normal third heart sound. In persons who are between 20 and 30 years of age, the third heart sound becomes less common. By 30 years of age, most men have lost S$_3$, although some women still retain it.

Origin of S_3

How S_3 is generated has been controversial. Recent studies indicate that S_3 (which occurs at the end of rapid early diastolic filling of the ventricle, when relaxation is over) is caused by a sudden intrinsic limitation of the longitudinal expansion of the ventricular wall. The resulting abrupt jerk is transmitted to the skin surface, and the low-frequency vibrations are perceived as S_3.

Listening for S_3

A normal S_3 increases and decreases in amplitude with respiration (Figure 8-1) and is usually loudest during inspiration (Figure 8-2). To hear S_3, the

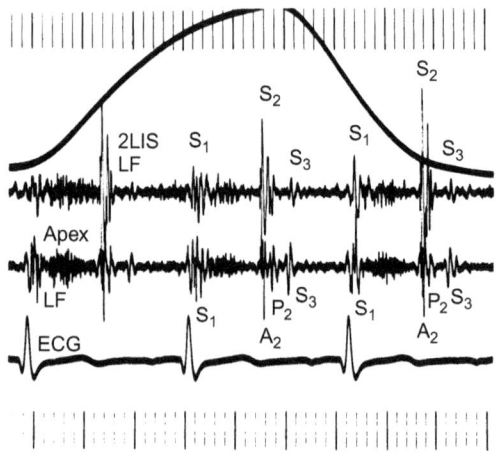

FIGURE 8-1. Third heart sound. Note that S_3 is louder over the apex during inspiration **(center)** than during expiration **(right)**. **2LIS,** Second left intercostal space; **LF,** low frequencies. (From Nadas AS, Fyler DC: **Pediatric cardiology,** ed 3, Philadelphia, 1972, WB Saunders. Copyright AS Nadas.)

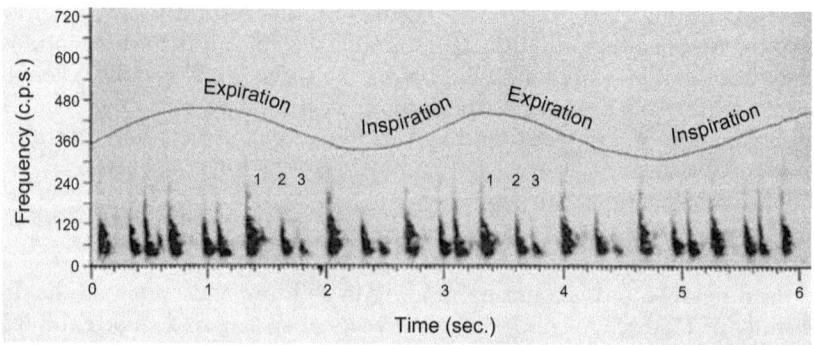

FIGURE 8-2. Spectral phonocardiogram of a third heart sound. Note that S_3 is louder on inspiration and that its frequency (pitch) is lower than that of S_1 or S_2. **c.p.s.,** Cycles per second. (From McKusick VA: **Cardiovascular sound in health and disease,** Baltimore, 1958, Williams & Wilkins.)

examiner should auscultate while asking the subject to breathe normally. S_3 is best heard if the child is recumbent or lying on the left side. S_3 is not heard as well if the child is sitting or standing. A left ventricular S_3 is loudest at the apex or just medial to the apex (Figure 8-3) and is increased by exercise, pressure on the abdomen, or lifting the legs. A right ventricular S_3 is loudest at the fourth intercostal space around the left sternal edge.

Pathologic Conditions Associated With S_3

S_3 of a normal amplitude is found in healthy children. S_3 of unusually high amplitude or high pitch, particularly if the sound is palpable, may indicate underlying heart failure or a hyperdynamic heart, stimulated to overwork by excitement, anemia, or a large left-to-right shunt. In a child with a rapid heart rate it may be difficult to differentiate S_3 from a summation gallop (S_3 and S_4 together) and from the middiastolic rumble heard at the apex in a large ventricular septal defect or patent ductus arteriosus.

THE FOURTH HEART SOUND

The term **fourth heart sound** may be used interchangeably with the terms **atrial sound, atrial gallop,** and **presystolic gallop.** Although a normal S_4 is sometimes found in a vigorously trained athlete with left atrial physiologic hypertrophy or in an elderly person, S_4 is not a normal finding in a child.

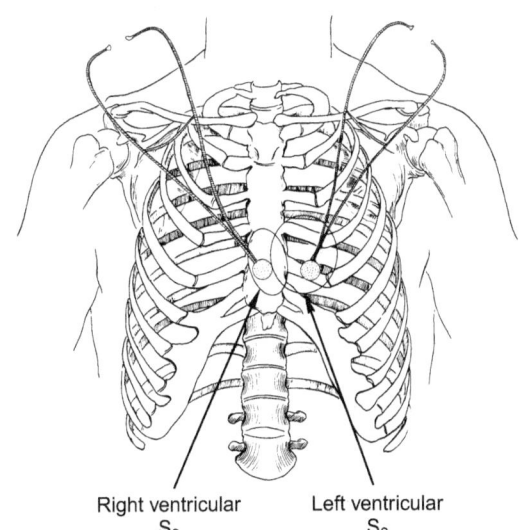

Right ventricular
S_3

Left ventricular
S_3

FIGURE 8-3. The third heart sound (S_3) is loudest at the apex or just medial to the apex.

Origin of S₄

The fourth heart sound is generated by vibrations resulting from atrial contraction. Indeed, S_4 corresponds with the A wave on the apexcardiogram (Figure 8-4) and the jugular venous pulse (Figure 8-5), both of which reflect atrial contraction. S_4 may be generated by either left or right atrial contraction.

Listening for S₄

S_4 is low-pitched (40 to 60 Hz), although the pitch tends to increase with the amplitude of the sound. Usually S_4 is not as loud as S_1, but it may

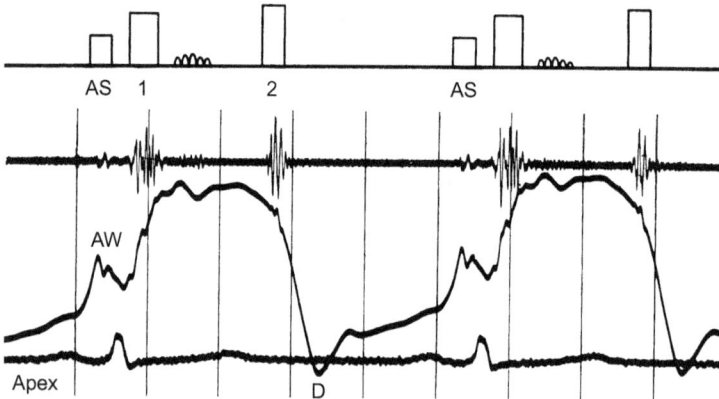

FIGURE 8-4. Apexcardiogram **(middle curve)** and phonocardiogram **(upper curve)** on a patient with a fourth heart sound (atrial sound [**AS**]). Note the prominent atrial wave **(AW)** on the apexcardiogram and its correspondence with the fourth heart sound (AS) on the phonocardiogram. The mitral valve opens at the **D** point. (From Ravin A, Craddock LD, Wolf PS et al: **Auscultation of the heart,** ed 3, Chicago, 1977, Year Book.)

FIGURE 8-5. Jugular venous pulse **(JVP)** and phonocardiograms of a patient with a fourth heart sound (S_4). Note that S_4 corresponds with the **a** wave of the jugular venous pulse. The phonocardiograms were made at the third and fourth left intercostal spaces (**3LIS** and **4LIS**), and the machine was set to be most sensitive to low frequencies **(LF)**. (From Nadas AS, Fyler DC: **Pediatric cardiology,** ed 3, Philadelphia, 1972, WB Saunders. Copyright AS Nadas.)

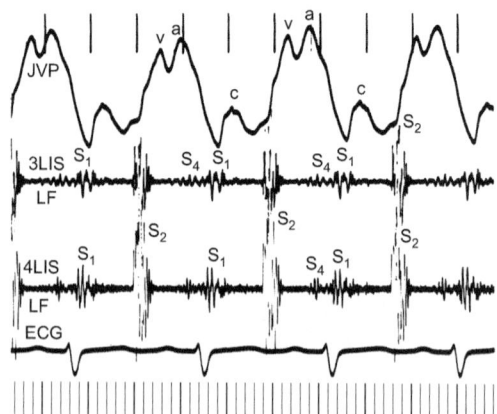

occasionally be louder. Because of the low pitch of S$_4$, the examiner should employ the bell of the stethoscope when listening for S$_4$. The bell should be applied lightly to the chest, in a very quiet room. S$_4$ is easiest to hear when the child is recumbent and may be more prominent after mild exercise. Sitting up and standing tend to diminish S$_4$. The Valsalva maneuver (expiring against a closed glottis) also reduces the amplitude of S$_4$, although it increases immediately afterward.

A left atrial fourth sound is best heard over the apex and is loudest on expiration. A split S$_1$ may also be audible at the apex in children, but it is louder at the lower left sternal border. A click is higher in pitch.

A right atrial fourth heart sound is loudest along the left sternal border and is increased by inspiration. The normally split S$_1$, also heard in this area, can be distinguished from S$_4$ by the fact that S$_1$ splitting is most prominent on expiration. Sometimes, when loud and widely separated from S$_1$, S$_4$ may sound like a short murmur (the atrial systolic murmur) or be confused with the presystolic murmur of mitral stenosis.

Pathologic Conditions Associated With S$_4$

Usually originating in the right atrium in children, S$_4$ is associated with the following disorders, all characterized by high right atrial pressure:

1. Primary pulmonary hypertension
2. Pure pulmonic stenosis
3. Ebstein's anomaly, in which a third heart sound is also often present, producing the characteristic "quadruple rhythm" associated with this lesion
4. Tricuspid atresia
5. Total anomalous pulmonary venous return (Figure 8-6)
6. Complete heart block

A left-sided S$_4$ may be heard in children with severe left ventricular disease, such as that caused by aortic stenosis or coarctation of the aorta.

SUMMATION GALLOP

When S$_3$ and S$_4$ occur at the same time, a single sound is produced that is often more intense than either component. This single sound is called a **summation gallop** (Figure 8-7). The summation gallop, apart from the almost pathognomonic quadruple rhythm of Ebstein's anomaly, is the most important and certainly the most common type of gallop heard in pediatric patients. A summation gallop is a pathologic finding commonly associated with heart failure.

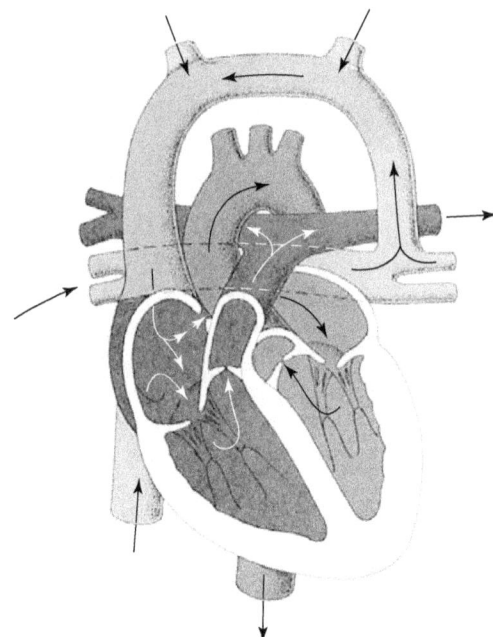

FIGURE 8-6. Total anomalous pulmonary venous connection (supracardiac, showing pulmonary veins connected to the left innominate vein). The presence of an atrial septal defect is necessary to allow blood to reach the left side of the heart. (From Foster R, Hunsberger MM, Anderson JT: **Family-centered nursing care of children,** Philadelphia, 1989, WB Saunders.)

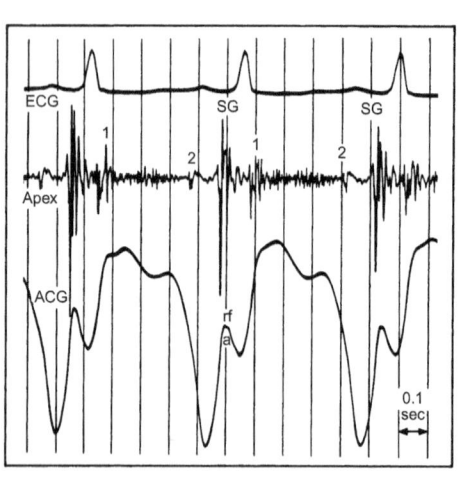

A

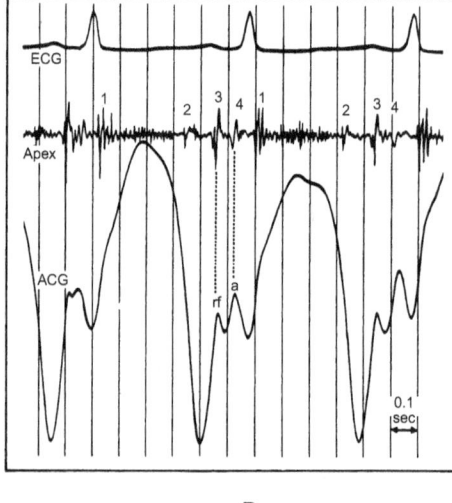

B

FIGURE 8-7. Summation gallop in a 13-year-old boy with aortic stenosis. **A** shows the loud summation gallop **(SG)** at the point at which the **a** wave and the peak of the rapid-filling waves of the ACG coincide. **B** was taken immediately after slowing of the rate with carotid sinus pressure. The third and fourth heart sounds have been separated and each is softer than its composite above. **ACG,** Apex cardiogram; **rf,** rapid-filling wave. (From Tavel ME: **Clinical phonocardiography and external pulse recording,** ed 4, Chicago, 1985, Year Book.)

BIBLIOGRAPHY

Alley RD, van Mierop LHS: Diseases—congenital anomalies. In Yonkman FF, editor: **Heart: the Ciba collection of medical illustrations,** Summit, NJ, 1969, Ciba-Geigy.

Braunwald E, Perloff JK: Physical examination of the heart and circulation. In Braunwald E, Zipes DP, Libby P, editors: **Heart disease,** ed 6, Philadelphia, 2001, WB Saunders.

McKusick VA: **Cardiovascular sound in health and disease,** Baltimore, 1958, Williams & Wilkins.

O'Rourke RA, Shaver JA, Silverman ME: The history, physical examination, and cardiac auscultation. In Fuster V, Alexander RW, O'Rourke RA, editors: **Hurst's the heart,** New York, 2001, McGraw-Hill.

Ozawa Y, Smith D, Craige E: Origin of the third heart sound. I. Studies in dogs, **Circulation** 67:393, 1983.

Ozawa Y, Smith D, Craige E: Origin of the third heart sound. II. Studies in human subjects, **Circulation** 67:399, 1983.

Perloff JK: **The clinical recognition of congenital heart disease,** ed 4, Philadelphia, 1994, WB Saunders.

Ravin A, Craddock LD, Wolf PS et al: **Auscultation of the heart,** ed 3, Chicago, 1977, Year Book.

Tavel ME: **Clinical phonocardiography and external pulse recording,** ed 4, Chicago, 1985, Year Book.

Tilkian AA, Conover MB: **Understanding heart sounds and murmurs,** ed 3, Philadelphia, 2001, WB Saunders.

Chapter 9

Other Systolic and Diastolic Sounds

In addition to the four heart sounds (S_1, S_2, S_3, and S_4), other sounds may occur in either systole or diastole. Extra sounds heard in systole include the **midsystolic click** and the **ejection sounds** (or clicks). In diastole, an opening snap may be audible.

SYSTOLIC CLICKS

Clicks arising from within the heart are one of the least easily recognized auscultatory findings in children. Both aortic and pulmonic ejection clicks, which are commonly missed on clinical examination, are important manifestations of aortic or pulmonic stenosis. Of the nonejection clicks, the midsystolic click of mitral leaflet prolapse is indicative of one of the most common congenital heart malformations. Yet many clinicians admit that they are unaware of this sound or have rarely heard it.

Differentiating Clicks From Other Sounds

Clicks are snappy, sharp sounds differing in pitch and duration from normal heart sounds (Figure 9-1). As mentioned, they are often missed on auscultation and, when detected, may be close enough to the first heart sound to be confused with a split S_1 or other extra sound. The midsystolic click of mitral valve prolapse may also be mistaken for physiologic splitting of the first heart sound or may be thought to be an innocent extracardiac sound or a third heart sound. In addition, in 25% of patients, mitral leaflet prolapse generates multiple clicks, which occasionally sound like a friction rub (see Chapter 11).

The quality and timing of the clicking sound and the presence or absence of associated murmurs allow the click to be correctly identified. For instance, the third heart sound is heard in the first third of diastole, whereas the

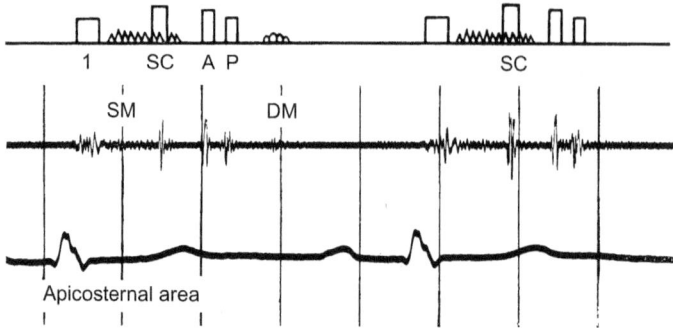

FIGURE 9-1. Systolic click. This patient had an atrial septal defect, and the midsystolic click *(SC)* was heard on only one occasion. The patient had been seen several other times and no systolic click was heard. The click was most evident on expiration. It was not heard in the pulmonic or aortic region but was confined to the area between the apex and the left border of the sternum. Note the split second heart sound characteristic of atrial septal defect. In this condition, the split second heart sound is often evident at the apex, despite the absence of an accentuated pulmonic sound. A middiastolic murmur *(DM)* is commonly heard in the apicosternal region in patients with atrial septal defects. **A,** Aortic component of second heart sound; **P,** pulmonic component of second heart sound; *SM,* systolic murmur. (From Ravin A, Craddock D, Wolf PS et al: *Auscultation of the heart,* ed 3, Chicago, 1977, Year Book.)

midsystolic click is heard in midsystole. The following technique helps to discern a click and differentiate it from other sounds:

1. **Analyze the sound.** The click is not very loud or long and is usually localized to a small area around the apex.
2. **Auscultate the patient in both standing and supine positions.** Standing promotes mitral valve prolapse by reducing left ventricular volume but does not affect a friction rub.
3. **Auscultate in a quiet room.** Because clicks are not very loud, they may be missed in the presence of background noise.
4. **Use the diaphragm of the stethoscope.** The diaphragm is best for hearing high-pitched sounds. Only relatively loud clicks can be heard with the bell.
5. **Make the search for clicks a routine part of every heart examination.** At least half the children with mitral leaflet prolapse have a click as the only auscultatory feature. The other characteristic feature, late systolic murmur, is discussed in Chapter 11.

MIDSYSTOLIC CLICK
Identifying the Midsystolic Click

The difficulty of hearing a midsystolic click, and the care needed to do so, were demonstrated in an interesting experiment by Dr. Dan McNamara of Children's Hospital in Houston, Texas. A 12-year-old girl with two midsystolic clicks was used as a test subject. The clicks were audible in a small area around the apex of the heart, were heard best while the girl was standing, and were inaudible while she was lying on her back or left side. She also had an innocent aortic vibratory murmur, which was best heard while she was lying on her back. There was no mitral murmur in any position. Therefore, the two midsystolic clicks were the only auscultatory clues to mitral valve leaflet prolapse, which was confirmed on an echocardiogram.

Dr. McNamara asked 11 physicians to examine the child. Dr. McNamara did not reveal whether an abnormality was present, and he remained in the room to observe each examiner's technique and to guard against the knowledgeable girl's revealing the correct diagnosis. All 11 examiners heard the innocent aortic vibratory murmur. Six, distracted by the murmur, did not hear the clicks. Of the five who did hear the clicks, four heard them while the girl was standing. Only one heard the clicks while the girl was seated.

The disparity in the findings of the 11 examiners emphasizes the importance of auscultating while the patient is standing as well as sitting and lying down. The importance of this point cannot be overemphasized. The child should be examined with the bell and diaphragm of the stethoscope, from apex to upper right sternal border and back again.

Echocardiography in the Diagnosis of Mitral Valve Prolapse

The prolapse of the posterior mitral valve leaflet is a characteristic echocardiographic finding in mitral valve prolapse. This echocardiographic finding is commonly overread, and the diagnosis of a prolapsed mitral valve should be made mainly on physical examination and only confirmed by echocardiography. In general, the diagnosis should not be made if abnormal heart sounds are not audible.

Management of Mitral Valve Prolapse

The diagnosis of mitral valve prolapse may not necessarily warrant intervention. If the echocardiogram shows a normal-looking mitral valve and no insufficiency, prolapse by itself may not be associated with adverse sequelae. There is also debate about whether a click, if not associated with a murmur of mitral insufficiency, is significant and warrants antibiotic prophylaxis against bacterial endocarditis.

AORTIC EJECTION SOUNDS
Origin and Nature of Aortic Ejection Sounds

Aortic ejection sounds are high-frequency clicks heard early in systole, just after the Q wave of the electrocardiogram (Figure 9-2). These sounds are most commonly associated with a congenital aortic stenosis, a deformed or bicuspid aortic valve (the normal aortic valve has three cusps), or rheumatic heart disease. The valve must be mobile to generate a sound. Heavy calcification impairs valve mobility and obliterates the ejection sound.

Listening for Aortic Ejection Sounds

Aortic ejection sounds are readily audible over the entire precordium and are particularly loud at the apex. Their intensity does not vary with respiration. They are best heard with the diaphragm of the stethoscope (see Figures 9-2 and 9-3).

PULMONIC EJECTION SOUNDS

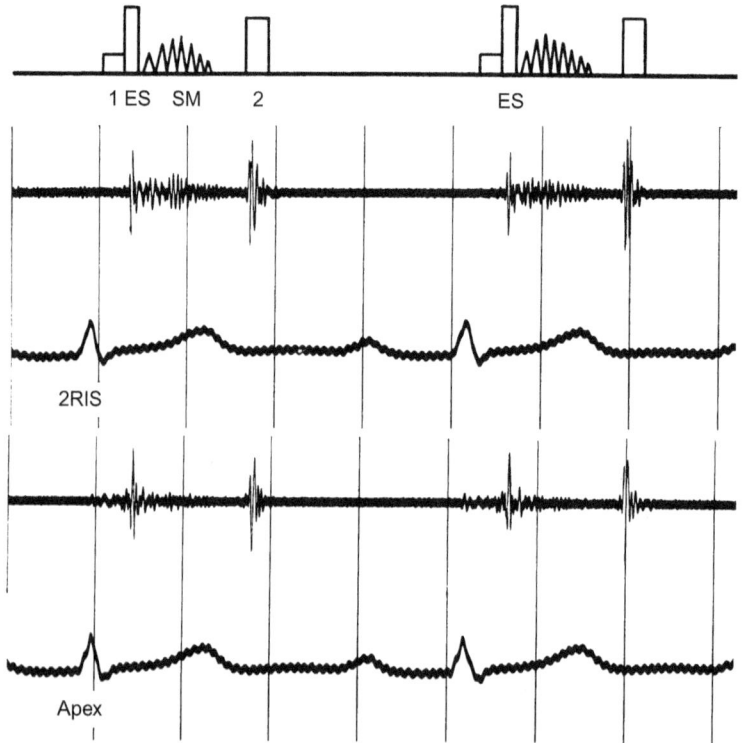

FIGURE 9-2. Aortic ejection sound *(ES)* in a patient with mild congenital aortic stenosis. This sound was heard well at the apex and at the second right intercostal space. Its intensity was not appreciably affected by respiration. The first sound was faint, especially in the aortic area. A rough systolic murmur *(SM)* of maximum intensity at the second right intercostal space was present. The murmur was faint at the apex. *2RIS,* Second right intercostal space. (From Ravin A, Craddock D, Wolf PS et al: *Auscultation of the heart,* ed 3, Chicago, 1977, Year Book.)

Origin and Nature of Pulmonic Ejection Sounds

Pulmonic ejection sounds, like aortic ejection sounds, are caused by valve abnormalities, such as congenital stenosis. Pulmonary hypertension and dilatation of the pulmonary artery also produce pulmonic ejection sounds. For example, one can hear the ejection sounds during the postoperative period in a patient who has undergone surgical correction of an atrial septal defect.

Listening for Pulmonic Ejection Sounds

Pulmonic ejection sounds are usually heard only over the upper left sternal border. They occur earlier in systole than aortic ejection sounds, after the Q wave of the electrocardiogram. A characteristic feature of the pulmonic ejection sound is that the sound is loudest during expiration (Figure 9-4).

Unlike the midsystolic click of mitral valve prolapse, aortic and pulmonic ejection sounds, especially when secondary to aortic stenosis or pulmonic stenosis, are rarely heard in the absence of murmurs. This helps differentiate them from a split S_1.

SYSTOLIC WHOOPS

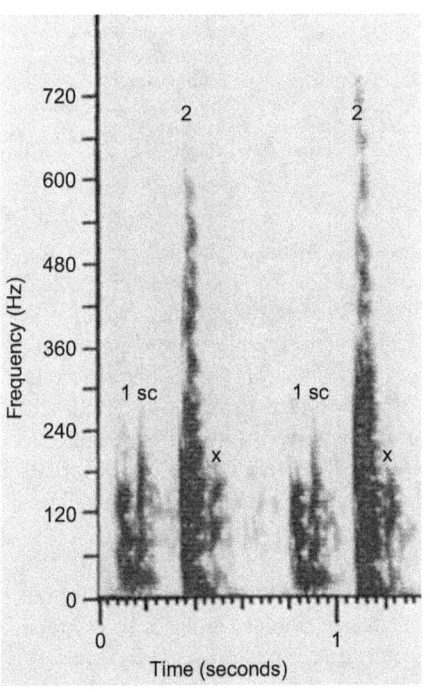

FIGURE 9-3. Sound spectrogram of early systolic click (*sc*, ejection sound). Note that the click is sharply separated from the first heart sound in the upper frequencies but blends with the first heart sound in the lower frequencies. Therefore, the diaphragm of the stethoscope, which passes the higher frequencies while filtering out the lower frequencies, is best for hearing the click. The spectrogram also shows a short systolic murmur and an early diastolic sound (*x*). (From McKusick VA: *Cardiovascular sound in health and disease*, Baltimore, 1958, Williams & Wilkins.)

Origin and Nature of Systolic Whoops

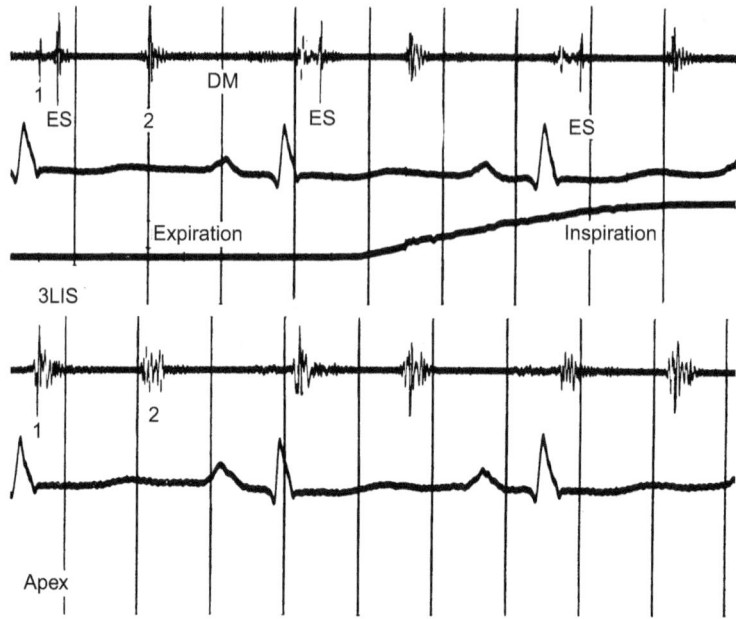

FIGURE 9-4. Pulmonic ejection sound *(ES)* in pulmonary hypertension with dilatation of pulmonary artery. This sound is best heard in the second and third left intercostal spaces and is loudest in expiration. It has a clicking quality. The auscultatory impression is very similar to that of a split first sound with a loud second component. The sound is not heard at the apex *(lower tracing)*. A high-pitched diastolic murmur *(DM)* is present *(upper tracing)* and is produced by pulmonary regurgitation. As is generally true, a high-pitched murmur is much more evident to the ear than on a tracing. *3LIS,* Third left intercostal space. (From Ravin A, Craddock D, Wolf PS et al: *Auscultation of the heart,* ed 3, Chicago, 1977, Year Book.)

A whoop is a loud, variable, musical sound audible over the apex in the latter part of systole. The whoop may be preceded by a systolic click, also variable in intensity. A whoop is sometimes called a **honk,** because it resembles the cry of a goose (Figure 9-5). Late systolic whoops and honks are associated with true mitral valve prolapse. Innocent vibratory murmurs may also have a honking quality, as may occasional murmurs of subaortic stenosis and closing ventricular septal defects with aneurysms of the ventricular septum. Echocardiography may be needed to distinguish between the innocent vibratory murmur and a honk associated with a structural abnormality.

Most whoops are generated by the mitral valve as it balloons into the left atrium during systole. The whoop often results from a pathologic change in the mitral valve. Indeed, long-term follow-up reveals that some whoops become systolic murmurs after a decade or more. Of eight recently studied patients who had whoops, five had systolic mitral regurgitation. Rarely, the

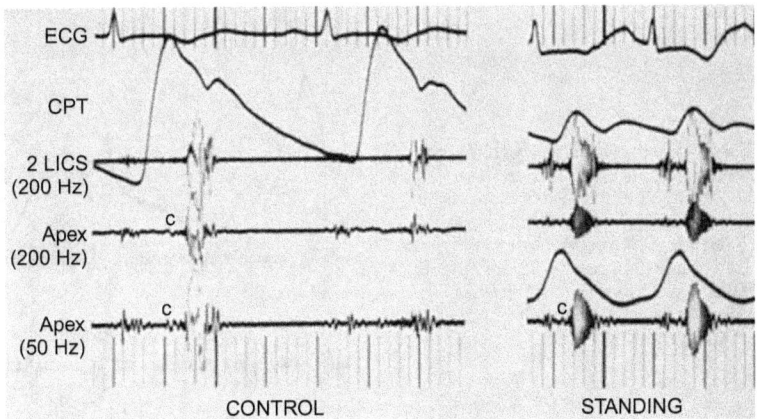

FIGURE 9-5. Systolic honk. With the child supine (control) there is a midsystolic click *(c)* and an intermittent late systolic honk. When the child is standing, the click and honk occur earlier in systole, and the honk increases in intensity. *2LICS,* Second left intercostal space; *Apex,* apexcardiogram; *CPT,* carotid pulse tracing. (From Felner JM, Harwood S, Mond H et al: Systolic honks in young children, *Am J Cardiol* 40:206-211, 1977.)

tricuspid valve can also cause a whoop.

Management of Whoops

Children with whoops resulting from a mitral valve abnormality, as determined by detection of a coexisting midsystolic click or by echocardiography, and their parents should be advised of the necessity of prophylaxis against subacute bacterial endocarditis.

OPENING SNAP OF THE MITRAL VALVE
Origin of the Mitral Opening Snap

During diastole, the normal mitral valve opens silently. In patients with rheumatic heart disease, in whom the valve leaflets are distorted or thickened, a characteristic high-pitched snapping sound (from the opening snap of the mitral valve) may be heard (Figure 9-6).

Listening for the Mitral Opening Snap

The opening snap occurs after the second heart sound. Although it radiates widely and is audible over most of the precordium, the snap is best heard over the midprecordium at the fourth left intercostal space.

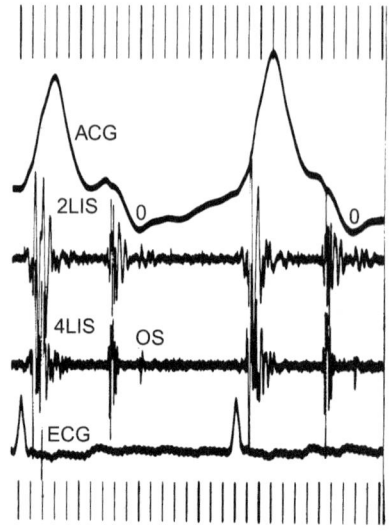

FIGURE 9-6. Opening snap in a patient with mitral stenosis. Upper tracing is an apexcardiogram. Note that the opening snap *(OS)* corresponds to the O point on the apexcardiogram. **ACG,** Apexcardiogram; *2LIS,* second left intercostal space; *4LIS,* fourth left intercostal space. (From Nadas AS, Fyler DC: *Pediatric cardiology,* ed 3, Philadelphia, 1972, WB Saunders. Copyright AS Nadas.)

Differentiating the Mitral Opening Snap From Other Sounds

Split S_2

When heard over the pulmonary area (second and third left intercostal spaces near the sternum), the opening snap may be mistaken for a **split second heart sound.** One can differentiate between the two by focusing careful attention on the components of the second heart sound. If an opening snap is present, three sounds should be audible during inspiration: A_2, P_2, and the opening snap. During expiration, only two components are heard: S_2 and the opening snap. The three components are sometimes referred to as a **trill** and result from the opening snap plus the normally widened split of A_2 and P_2 during inspiration (Figure 9-7).

Atrial Septal Defect

Sometimes the opening snap of mitral stenosis may be confused with the widely split fixed second heart sound of patients with atrial septal defect. The likelihood of confusion is increased if the middiastolic murmur of mitral stenosis is mistaken for the diastolic flow rumble of atrial septal defect. To differentiate between the two, the examiner should pay close attention to the respiratory variation of the second heart sound over the pulmonary area, where A_2 and P_2 are audible. In atrial septal defect, respiration has no effect on the wide splitting of S_2. In mitral stenosis, the double sound audible during expiration (S_2 plus the opening snap) changes to a trill or triple sound during inspiration (A_2, P_2, and the opening snap). Also, the diastolic flow murmur of atrial septal defect originates from the tricuspid valve and is therefore heard best over the third intercostal space at the lower left sternal border, whereas the diastolic murmur of mitral stenosis is loudest at the apex.

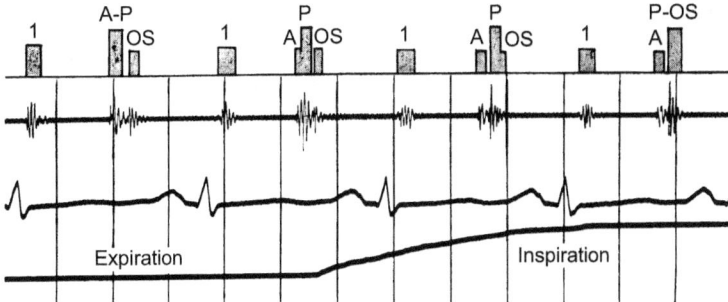

FIGURE 9-7. Opening snap of mitral valve. In this patient, the opening snap *(OS)* is quite close to the aortic *(A)* and pulmonic *(P)* second sound on expiration, and the splitting that occurs on inspiration is enough to place the pulmonic second sound on top of the opening snap. The two sounds heard on expiration are thus (1) the combined aortic and pulmonic second sounds and (2) the opening snap. On inspiration, the two sounds are (1) the aortic second sound and (2) the combined pulmonic second sound and opening snap. (From Ravin A, Craddock D, Wolf PS et al: *Auscultation of the heart,* ed 3, Chicago, 1977, Year Book.)

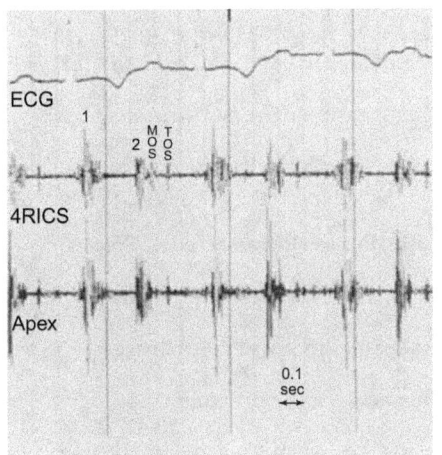

FIGURE 9-8. Combined mitral and tricuspid opening snaps *(MOS and TOS, respectively)* in a patient with stenosis of both valves. Both snaps are noted at the fourth right intercostal space *(4RICS).* (From Tavel ME: *Clinical phonocardiography and external pulse recording,* ed 4, Chicago, 1985, Year Book.)

The opening snap of the mitral valve is uncommon in pediatric patients, because children rarely have pure mitral stenosis or mitral stenosis resulting from rheumatic fever. Mitral and tricuspid insufficiency are much more common.

OPENING SNAP OF THE TRICUSPID VALVE
Origin and Nature of the Tricuspid Opening Snap

The tricuspid opening snap is caused by tricuspid stenosis, which may occur postoperatively or as part of the hypoplastic right heart syndrome. If tricuspid stenosis is the result of rheumatic heart disease, mitral stenosis is generally an associated finding (Figure 9-8).

Listening for the Tricuspid Opening Snap

The tricuspid opening snap is not commonly detected. The snap is loudest at the lower end of the sternum and the lower right sternal border. It occurs only 0.02 second after the mitral opening snap, which tends to obscure it.

BIBLIOGRAPHY

Behar VS, Whalen RE, McIntosh HD: Ballooning mitral valve in patients with the "precordial honk" or "whoop," **Am J Cardiol** 20:789, 1967.

Bisset GS, Schwartz DC, Meyer RA et al: Clinical spectrum and long-term follow up of isolated mitral valve prolapse in 119 children, **Circulation** 62:423-429, 1980.

Braunwald E, Perloff JK: Physical examination of the heart and circulation. In Braunwald E, Zipes DP, Libby P, editors: **Heart disease,** ed 6, Philadelphia, 2001, WB Saunders.

Dayem M, Wasfi RM, Bentall HH et al: Investigation and treatment of constrictive pericarditis, **Thorax** 22:242, 1967.

Felner JE, Harwood S, Mond H et al: Systolic honks in young children, **Am J Cardiol** 40:206-211, 1977.

Friedman WF, Silverman N: Congenital heart disease in infancy and childhood. In Braunwald E, Zipes DP, Libby P, editors: **Heart disease,** ed 6, Philadelphia, 2001, WB Saunders.

Giardina A: Resurgence of acute rheumatic fever, **N Engl J Med** 317:507-508, 1987.

Liebman J: Diagnosis and management of heart murmurs in children, **Pediatr Rev** 3:321-329, 1982.

McNamara DG: Idiopathic benign mitral leaflet prolapse. The pediatrician's view, **Am J Dis Child** 136:152-156, 1982.

O'Rourke RA, Shaver JA, Silverman ME: The history, physical examination, and cardiac auscultation. In Fuster V, Alexander RW, O'Rourke RA, editors: **Hurst's the heart,** New York, 2001, McGraw-Hill.

Ravin A, Craddock LD, Wolf PS et al: **Auscultation of the heart,** ed 3, Chicago, 1977, Year Book.

Silberner J: Mysterious return of a childhood scourge, **US News & World Report,** p 64, Aug 31, 1987.

Tavel ME: **Clinical phonocardiography and external pulse recording,** ed 4, Chicago, 1985, Year Book.

Tilkian AA, Conover MB: **Understanding heart sounds and murmurs,** ed 3, Philadelphia, 2001, WB Saunders.

Veasy LG, Wiedmeier SE, Orsmond GS et al: Resurgence of acute rheumatic fever in the intermountain area of the United States, **N Engl J Med** 316:421-427, 1987.

Chapter 10

General Characteristics of Murmurs

Murmurs are relatively long noises (compared with heart sounds) generated by the turbulent flow of blood in the cardiovascular system. The existence of abnormal connections between the chambers of the heart and two valvular conditions, **stenosis** and **regurgitation,** are the causes of most cardiac murmurs. The character of a murmur is determined by the velocity of blood flow and the vibration of surrounding structures.

ORIGIN OF MURMURS

Stenosis

Stenosis can be divided into two general categories. A narrowed or irregular valve that impedes blood flow is said to be **organically stenotic.** A valve is said to be **relatively stenotic** if (1) the valve itself is normal, but the chamber or vessel beyond is enlarged or (2) flow through a normal-sized orifice is increased. For example, a murmur is present in children with a patent ductus arteriosus or a ventricular septal defect that causes increased flow (the murmur of relative mitral stenosis) even though the valve itself is not stenotic.

Regurgitation

A valve that is incompetent and permits the backward flow of blood is said to be **regurgitant** or **insufficient.** Regurgitation may occur because of congenital or pathologically acquired deformities of the valve or supporting structures. For example, the cleft valve caused by an endocardial cushion defect is a congenitally acquired valve defect that causes regurgitation. An example of a pathologically acquired deformity is the damage resulting from subacute bacterial endocarditis, a chronic infection.

Deformities in the valve may be limited or extensive, and there may be thickening and shortening of the cusps and chordae tendineae. The valve ring may be dilated, and in the atrioventricular valves, ventricular dilatation may be so great that the chordae tendineae are too short to allow the valve edges to approximate. Regurgitation caused by deformed valve cusps is called **organic regurgitation.** Regurgitation through normal valve cusps is called **functional regurgitation.**

NATURE OF MURMURS

Murmurs are defined by their timing in the cardiac cycle, their loudness or intensity, and their pitch and quality. Each of these characteristics is discussed in the following sections.

Timing

Timing in the cardiac cycle is one of the criteria for classifying a murmur (Figure 10-1). A murmur is said to be **systolic** if it occurs between S_1 and S_2, and **diastolic** if it occurs between S_2 and S_1. Systolic murmurs may be further classified as early, mid, or late. A holosystolic murmur is heard throughout systole. Diastolic murmurs may also be classified as early, mid,

FIGURE 10-1. Classification of murmurs by timing. Note that a continuous murmur need not continue throughout diastole.

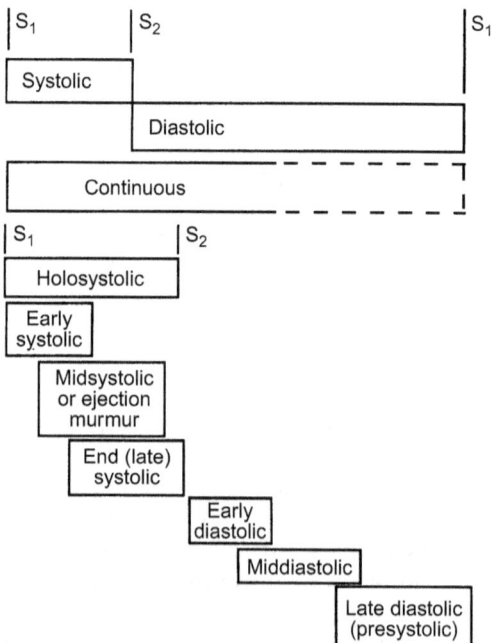

or late (presystolic). A **continuous murmur** begins in systole and continues into diastole.

Differentiating Systole From Diastole

At normal heart rates, systole is easily distinguished from diastole, because systole is shorter. When the heart rate is rapid, the differentiation between the two becomes more difficult, and the following technique may be of help:

1. **Observe the point of maximum impulse.** An apical impulse is visible during systole. Place the bell of the stethoscope over the point of maximum impulse and watch its motion.
2. **Inspect and palpate the carotid artery.** This method is used in adults but is difficult to perform in children and is not frequently employed in practice.

Loudness

Murmurs are graded in six steps according to loudness (intensity). This classification, first proposed by Freeman and Levine in 1933, is still in use.

Grade I. A grade I murmur is audible only with special concentration, is distinct but very faint, and is usually not heard during the first few seconds of listening.

Grade II. A grade II murmur is louder than a grade I murmur but still faint and not immediately audible.

Grade III. A grade III murmur is of intermediate intensity; it is prominent and louder than a grade II murmur and may be associated with a thrill.

Grade IV. A grade IV murmur is loud but still considered to be of intermediate intensity. It must be associated with a palpable vibration or thrill.

Grade V. A grade V murmur is very loud and is audible even with only one edge of the stethoscope against the chest wall. Grade V is associated with a palpable thrill.

Grade VI. A grade VI murmur is the loudest possible murmur; it is audible even when the stethoscope is not in contact with the chest wall and may be heard with the ear near the chest wall. It is associated with a palpable thrill.

The timing and loudness of murmurs may be indicated graphically (Figures 10-2 and 10-3). If a murmur begins softly and becomes louder, it is called a **crescendo murmur.** If it begins loudly and becomes softer, it is called a **decrescendo murmur.** A crescendo-decrescendo murmur is diamond shaped, increasing and then decreasing in loudness. Sometimes a crescendo-decrescendo murmur is also called an **ejection murmur.**

Pitch and Quality

The frequency composition of a murmur affects how it is perceived. The relation between pitch and quality of a murmur is shown in Figure 10-4. Occasionally a murmur has a musical quality, because it is composed of harmonics (see Chapters 2 and 4).

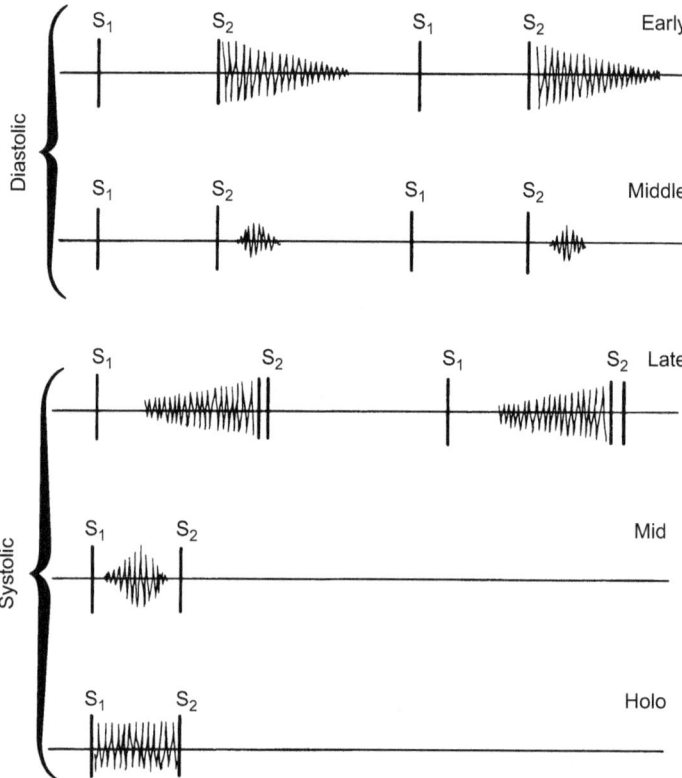

FIGURE 10-2. A method for recording heart sounds and murmurs. Loudness is indicated by the height of the block. The width of the block indicates duration.

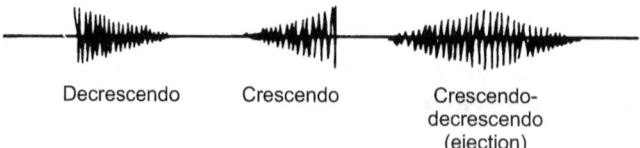

FIGURE 10-3. A method for recording waxing and waning of murmurs.

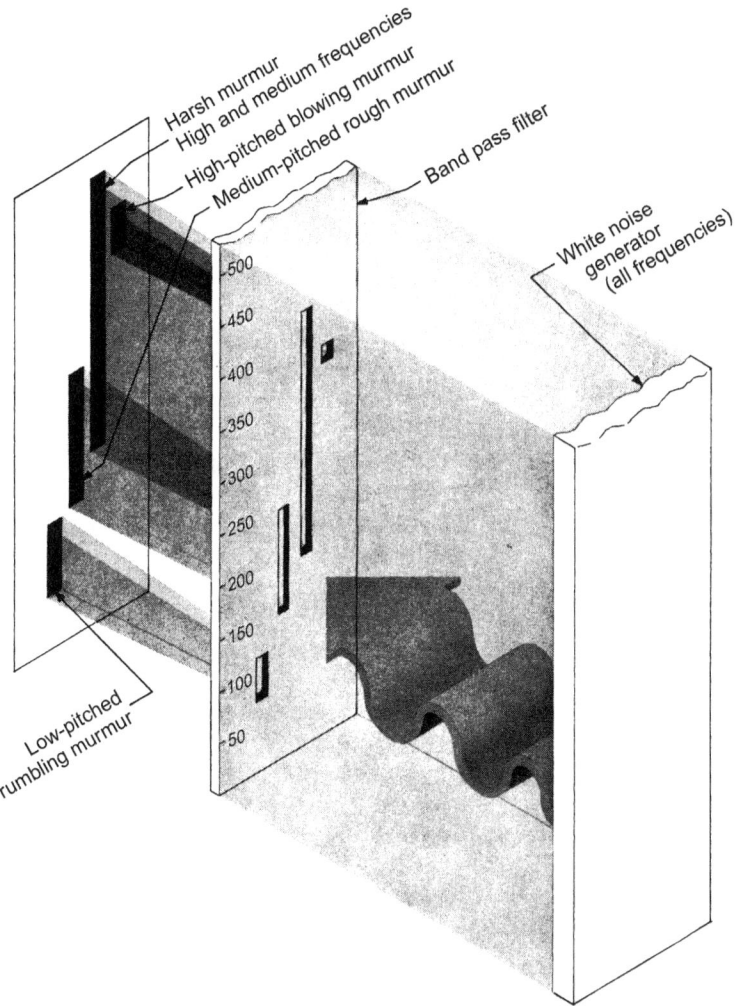

FIGURE 10-4. Frequency composition, pitch, and quality of murmurs. A sound containing all frequencies is called **white noise.** Produced by a white noise generator, this sound may be attenuated by a band pass filter to select the following frequencies, which simulate actual murmurs:
1. 180-460 Hz, high and medium frequencies, are perceived as a harsh murmur, similar to that of aortic or pulmonic stenosis.
2. 360 Hz, high frequency, is perceived as high-pitched and blowing, similar to the murmur of mitral and aortic regurgitation. Note that the murmurs of mitral regurgitation and aortic regurgitation do not always sound very similar.
3. 120-250 Hz, medium frequencies, are perceived as a medium-pitched and/or rough murmur.
4. 70-110 Hz, low frequencies, simulate a murmur that is low-pitched and rumbling.
(From Ravin A, Craddock LD, Wolf PS et al: **Auscultation of the heart,** ed 3, Chicago, 1977, Year Book.)

BIBLIOGRAPHY

Freeman AR, Levine SA: The clinical significance of the systolic murmur. A study of 1000 consecutive "non-cardiac" cases, **Ann Intern Med** 6:1371, 1933.

Ravin A, Craddock LD, Wolf PS et al: **Auscultation of the heart,** ed 3, Chicago, 1977, Year Book.

Tilkian AA, Conover MB: **Understanding heart sounds and murmurs,** ed 3, Philadelphia, 2001, WB Saunders.

Chapter 11

Systolic Murmurs

A systolic murmur is a common finding during the routine physical examination of a healthy infant or child. Differentiation between an innocent murmur and one that is a sign of heart disease presents a common diagnostic problem; the auscultatory findings needed to distinguish them are presented in this chapter. A murmur must be clearly defined, described, and categorized by precise criteria to identify children with a pathologic condition.

CLASSIFICATION OF SYSTOLIC MURMURS

Systolic murmurs are traditionally grouped into two principal categories: ejection murmurs and regurgitant (holosystolic) murmurs.

Ejection Murmurs

Ejection murmurs, or midsystolic murmurs, are heard in midsystole and are generated by the ejection of blood into the root of either the aorta or the pulmonary artery. The typical ejection murmurs are associated with stenosis of the aortic or pulmonic valves (Figure 11-1).

Regurgitant Murmurs

Regurgitant murmurs, or holosystolic murmurs, are audible throughout systole (i.e., they are **holosystolic**), and most are caused by incompetence of the atrioventricular valves. Because the pressure difference between the atria and ventricles is considerable throughout systole, a regurgitant murmur tends to have an even configuration (Figure 11-2) rather than the diamond shape of an ejection murmur.

Some cardiologists object to the traditional two-group classification of systolic murmurs. They point out that the murmur of a ventricular septal defect or patent ductus arteriosus has nothing to do with pressure differences between atria and ventricles, but rather between left ventricle and

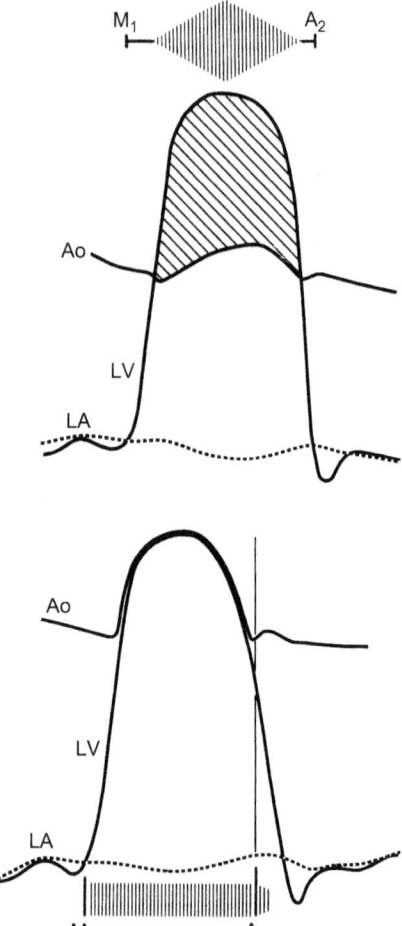

Figure 11-1. Midsystolic murmur in aortic stenosis, with pressure records from left ventricle **(LV)**, left atrium **(LA)**, and aorta **(Ao)**. In early systole, LV pressure rises swiftly and opens the aortic valve, whereupon ejection into the root of the aorta can begin. Only then does the midsystolic or ejection murmur start, peaking at the time of maximum gradient across the valve **(shaded area)**. At the end of systole, the falling pressure in the LV results in diminishing flow across the aortic valve, and the murmur fades away before A_2. (From Braunwald E: **Heart disease**, ed 6, Philadelphia, 2001, WB Saunders.)

Figure 11-2. Holosystolic murmur. In mitral regurgitation, LV pressure rises and immediately exceeds LA pressure. Thus, the regurgitant murmur begins with M_1, continues throughout systole, and may continue even slightly beyond A_2, because the falling pressure in the LV still exceeds that of the LA. **Ao,** Aorta; **LA,** left atrium; **LV,** left ventricle. (From Braunwald E: **Heart disease,** ed 6, Philadelphia, 2001, WB Saunders.)

right ventricle, or aorta and pulmonary artery. These cardiologists feel systolic murmurs are best described by quality (harsh, blowing, or musical), intensity (soft or loud), duration (short, long, or holosystolic), timing (early, mid, or late), location, and radiation.

INNOCENT SYSTOLIC MURMURS

The innocent systolic murmur, also called a **physiologic or benign murmur,** is a very common finding in children. Studies have shown that as many as 90% of healthy children may have an innocent murmur at some time. These murmurs may disappear quickly, or they may last for years. In either case, they must be differentiated from murmurs that indicate heart disease.

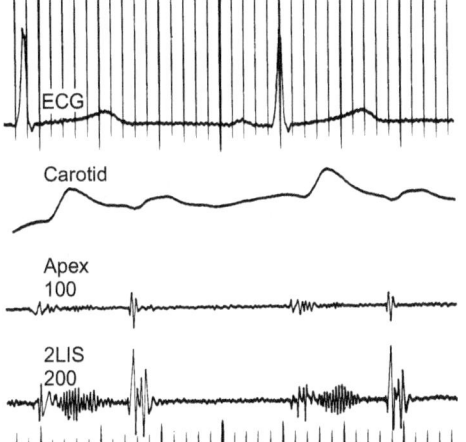

Figure 11-3. An innocent murmur at the second left intercostal space. Note the even, harmonic quality of the murmur heard only in the second left intercostal space **(2LIS)**. On auscultation this has a musical sound. (From Nadas AS, Fyler DC: **Pediatric cardiology,** ed 3, Philadelphia, 1972, WB Saunders. Copyright AS Nadas.)

Origin of the Innocent Systolic Murmur

A murmur can be detected in a normal person by placing an intracardiac phonocatheter at the root (origin) of the pulmonary artery or the aorta. Two anatomic features contribute to the generation of this innocent systolic murmur. First, the origins of the aorta and pulmonary artery are narrower than the ventricles ejecting blood into them, and second, both the aorta and the pulmonary artery arise from their respective ventricles at an angle.

These anatomic characteristics cause flowing blood to produce a noise analogous to the sound of water passing through a pipe. The murmur of water flowing through a pipe can be heard easily by putting your ear close to the pipe. If there is a partially closed valve, narrowing the orifice of the entering stream, the murmur becomes louder. The murmur becomes louder still over an angle in the pipe, where the flow is turbulent. In a child, especially a young one, the heart is very close to the chest wall, making it easy to hear the normal murmur on the surface of the chest.

Nature of the Innocent Systolic Murmur

Innocent systolic murmurs are ejection murmurs, usually of grade I to grade II intensity. They are augmented by exercise, anxiety, fever, or anemia and are best heard with the child in the supine position. Other signs and symptoms of heart disease are absent. These murmurs may be separated into two types, depending on the point of maximum intensity.

The first type is an innocent murmur with maximum intensity in the apicosternal region. This murmur, also called **Still's murmur,** may have a groaning, vibratory, or musical quality and can be heard over a wide area (Figure 11-3). A Still's murmur is audible in early systole to midsystole and has a crescendo-decrescendo form.

The second type is an innocent murmur with maximum intensity in the second left intercostal space (pulmonary area). This murmur is slightly harsh, occurs in early systole to midsystole, and is also crescendo-decrescendo in form. It may result from turbulent flow in the pulmonary artery.

INNOCENT EXTRACARDIAC MURMURS

Although most murmurs with a diastolic component are associated with a cardiac pathologic condition, the cervical venous hum and the mammary souffle, discussed in the following sections, are considered innocent.

Cervical Venous Hum

The cervical venous hum, a normal finding, is the most common continuous murmur found in children. Heard in both systole and diastole, the cervical venous hum is loudest during diastole (Figure 11-4). The humming noise is most audible in the supraclavicular space over the right internal jugular vein (Figure 11-5, **A**). The hum becomes less intense or even disappears when the child lies down or performs the Valsalva maneuver (forced expiration against a closed glottis). Gentle pressure on the internal jugular vein, just above the head of the clavicle, also causes it to disappear (Figure 11-5, **B**). The hum becomes louder when the head is rotated away from the side being examined.

Differentiation of the Cervical Venous Hum From Other Murmurs

If loud, the cervical venous hum may be transmitted to the anterior chest wall, where it may be mistaken for the murmur of patent ductus arteriosus or combined aortic stenosis and insufficiency. In addition to the

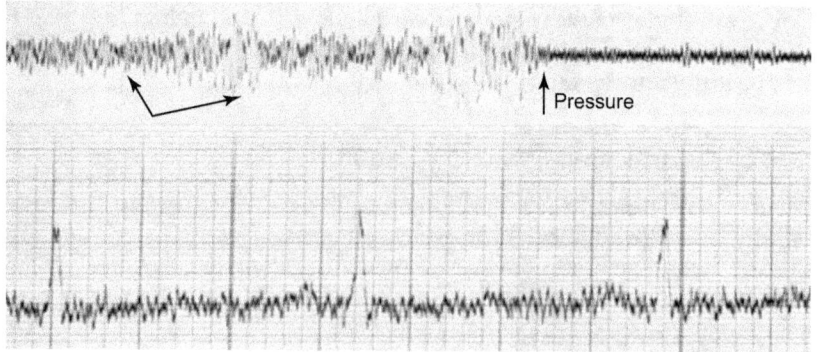

Figure 11-4. Venous hum in a healthy 24-year-old woman. The murmur is continuous. In the first cycle the diastolic component is louder **(paired arrows)**. Digital pressure on the right internal jugular vein **(vertical arrow)** completely obliterates the murmur. (From Perloff JK: **The clinical recognition of congenital heart disease**, ed 4, Philadelphia, 1994, WB Saunders.)

maneuvers already described, identification of diastolic accentuation helps to differentiate the cervical venous hum from other less common murmurs.

Mammary Souffle

The mammary souffle (the term **souffle** comes from the French word for "breath") is a continuous murmur heard only in lactating women and may be a consideration in an adolescent who is breast-feeding. The mammary souffle results from increased mammary blood flow and is heard over or just above the breasts. A mammary souffle is characteristically louder during systole (Figure 11-6) and may be obliterated by increasing the pressure on the stethoscope or compressing the tissue on both sides of the stethoscope. These maneuvers differentiate the mammary souffle from the murmurs of patent ductus arteriosus or combined aortic stenosis and insufficiency, which are unaffected by applied pressure.

Supraclavicular Arterial Bruit

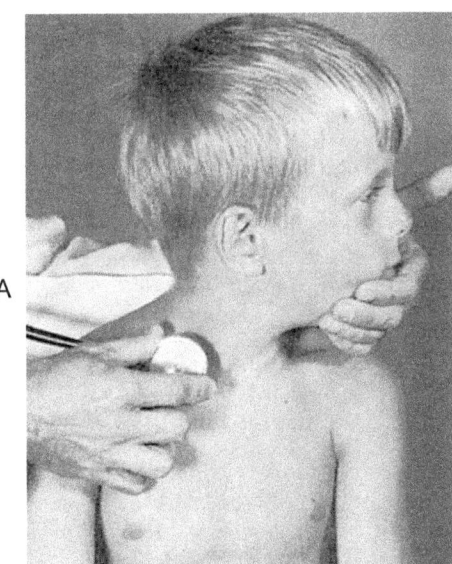
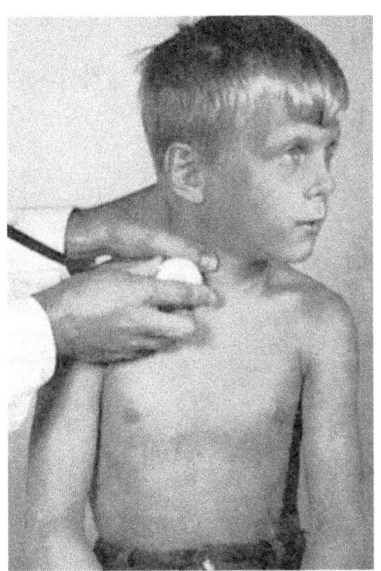

Figure 11-5. Maneuvers for eliciting or abolishing the venous hum. **A,** The bell of the stethoscope is applied to the medial aspect of the right supraclavicular fossa. The left hand grasps the patient's chin from behind and pulls it tautly to the left and upward.
B, Digital compression of the right internal jugular vein for obliteration of the hum. The head has returned to a more neutral position. (From Perloff JK: **The clinical recognition of congenital heart disease,** ed 4, Philadelphia, 1994, WB Saunders.)

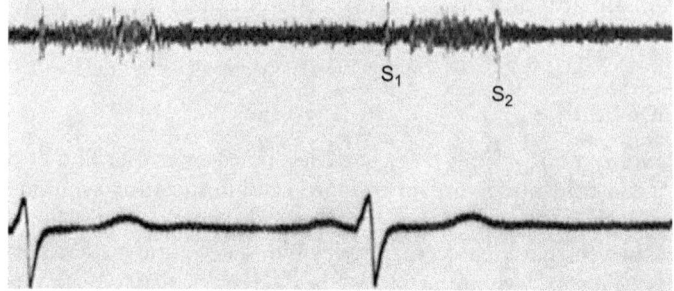

Figure 11-6. Continuous mammary souffle at the upper left chest in a normal 26-year-old lactating woman. The murmur is truly continuous but louder in systole and does **not** peak around the second heart sound (S_2). **S_1,** First heart sound. (From Perloff JK: **The clinical recognition of congenital heart disease,** ed 4, Philadelphia, 1994, WB Saunders.)

The supraclavicular bruit (the term **bruit** comes from the French word for "noise") is best heard just above the clavicles when the child is sitting. Bruits occur more commonly in anxious or anemic children. The bruit is short, starting in early systole and ending well before S_2. It may be produced by turbulence near the origin of the subclavian, innominate, and carotid arteries.

STRAIGHT BACK SYNDROME AND PECTUS EXCAVATUM

Children with straight back syndrome or pectus excavatum have a decreased anteroposterior (AP) diameter of the chest. In straight back syndrome, decreased AP diameter is caused by loss of the normal curvature of the upper thoracic spine. In pectus excavatum, reduced AP diameter is a result of the inward curvature of the sternum. Chest x-ray films demonstrate a leftward shift of the heart and increased angulation of the anterior ends of the middle and lower ribs (Figure 11-7).

Nature of the Murmur of Straight Back Syndrome and Pectus Excavatum

Children with straight back syndrome or pectus excavatum have a crescendo-decrescendo pulmonary murmur over the second and third left intercostal spaces, increased **inspiratory splitting** of S_2, occasional increased **expiratory splitting** of S_2 (which may be mistaken for the fixed splitting of S_2 heard in atrial septal defect), and splitting of S_1. There is also a marked systolic impulse in the left second and third intercostal spaces near the sternum.

Besides atrial septal defect, these findings may occasionally be mistaken for

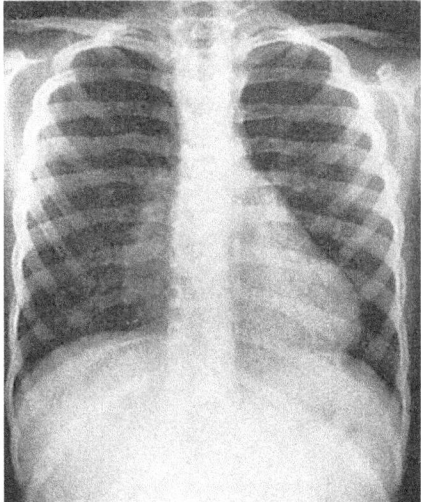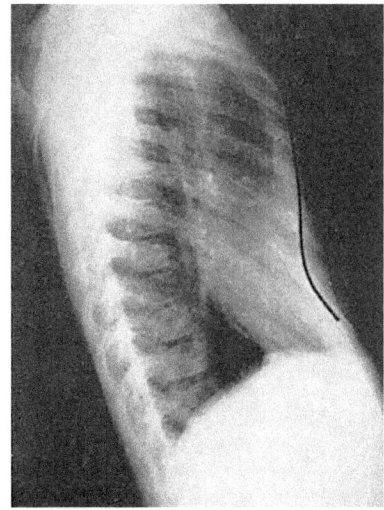

Figure 11-7. Typical radiographic findings in a 5-year-old boy with a pectus excavatum, demonstrating an absent right cardiac border and minimal deviation of the cardiac mass into the left hemithorax with angulation of the anterior ends of the middle and lower ribs. The chest is wide in the anteroposterior view and narrow in the lateral view. The lung fields are normal. (From Kendig E, Chernick V: **Disorders of the respiratory tract in children,** ed 4, Philadelphia, 1983, WB Saunders.)

mild pulmonic stenosis or dilatation of the pulmonary artery.

VENTRICULAR SEPTAL DEFECT

Origin of the Murmur of Ventricular Septal Defect

A ventricular septal defect is the most common lesion associated with a systolic murmur in children. A direct communication between the left and right ventricles, ventricular septal defect usually results from a single hole in the membranous portion of the interventricular septum (Figure 11-8). The direction of blood flow through a ventricular septal defect depends on pulmonary vascular outflow obstruction. If resistance is low, the flow is from left to right. If the patient has pulmonic stenosis, or if severe pulmonary hypertension has developed, the flow is from right to left.

Nature of the Murmur of Ventricular Septal Defect

In almost all affected children, the murmur of ventricular septal defect is discovered during the first year of life. The murmur is sometimes holo-systolic, although it commonly peaks during systole and may, in fact, be diamond shaped (Figure 11-9). Small ventricular septal defects are especially apt to have a diamond-shaped murmur. Faint or moderately loud murmurs are

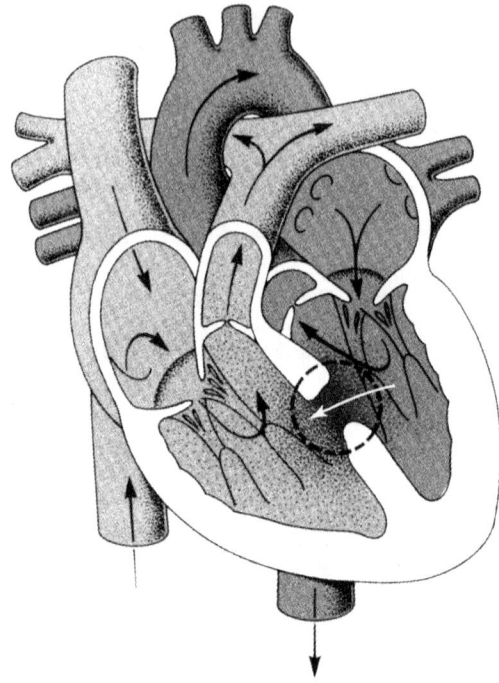

Figure 11-8. Ventricular septal defect. Abnormal flow is from left ventricle to right ventricle. (From Foster R, Hunsberger MM, Anderson JT: **Family-centered nursing care of children,** Philadelphia, 1990, WB Saunders.)

high-pitched, whereas loud murmurs are harsh. If the murmur is loud, a palpable thrill occurs.

The murmur is best heard with the stethoscope over the third or fourth intercostal space to the left of the sternum (Figure 11-10). Rarely, the murmur of a very high ventricular septal defect is loudest in the second left intercostal space when the patient is lying down. The transmission of the murmur is influenced by its intensity: very loud murmurs are audible over the entire precordium and over the back, although they may be difficult to hear in the neck.

If a large amount of blood is shunted from one side of the heart to the other, a rumbling apical middiastolic murmur may occur and is best heard at the apex in the left lateral decubitus position. The murmur is generated by increased blood flow through the mitral valve.

Pulmonary Hypertension

The development of pulmonary hypertension has a significant influence on the pathophysiologic consequences of ventricular septal defect. If pulmonary hypertension develops, the shunt becomes smaller and the murmur may become softer as pulmonary vascular resistance increases. When pulmonary hypertension is severe, the reduction in the left-to-right shunt may even be sufficient to cause the murmur to disappear. In addition, the

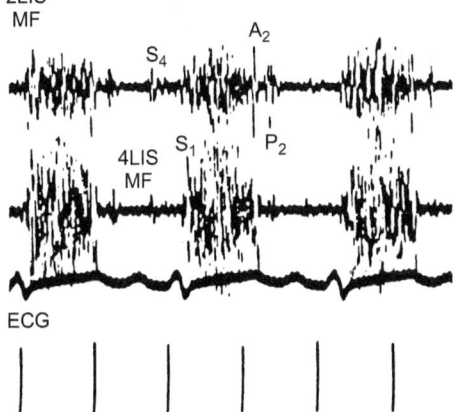

Figure 11-9. Systolic murmur of ventricular septal defect. Note that this murmur begins with the first heart sound, ends with the second heart sound, and is composed of high-frequency vibrations. Note also that the murmur is louder in the fourth left intercostal space **(4LIS)** than in the second left intercostal space **(2LIS). MF,** Medium frequency. (From Nadas AS, Fyler DC: **Pediatric cardiology,** ed 3, Philadelphia, 1972, WB Saunders. Copyright AS Nadas.)

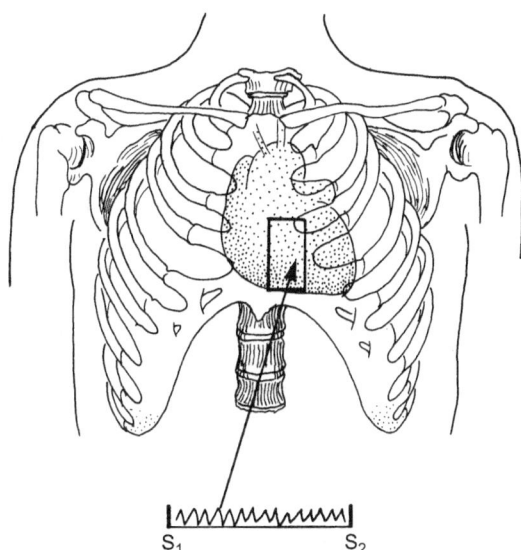

Figure 11-10. The murmur of ventricular septal defect (VSD) and where it is heard. A high membranous VSD may be loudest at the midleft sternal border. This murmur is often grade IV or louder and is easily audible over a wide area.

pulmonic component of the second heart sound becomes louder, and the splitting of A_2 and P_2 on inspiration diminishes or vanishes. If pulmonary hypertension is severe enough, a right-to-left shunt develops, and the patient becomes cyanotic. This is called **Eisenmenger syndrome.** To prevent the development of irreversible pulmonary hypertension, large shunts that persist beyond infancy must be closed.

Pulmonic insufficiency in association with a high pulmonary vascular resistance may cause a pulmonic ejection sound as well as a high-pitched early diastolic murmur along the left sternal border. The pulmonic murmur is best appreciated with the diaphragm of the stethoscope. As pressure on the right side of the heart increases, a right ventricular S_4 may become audible. In congestive heart failure, S_3 is also heard.

Additional Findings in Ventricular Septal Defect

A child with ventricular septal defect may have other congenital heart defects and associated chromosomal abnormalities (see Chapter 3). Some children with high defects may develop aortic insufficiency because of prolapse of a cusp of the aortic valve. In many children, the ventricular septal defect will eventually close spontaneously, in some even after the child is 4 or 5 years of age.

Differentiating Ventricular Septal Defect From Other Conditions

Patent Ductus Arteriosus

Ventricular septal defect can sometimes be confused with patent ductus arteriosus. It is especially difficult to separate ventricular septal defect with patent ductus arteriosus from patent ductus arteriosus alone, because the latter can cause a very harsh holosystolic murmur at the lower left sternal border. The following points may be of help:

1. The murmur of a large patent ductus is generally coarser than the murmur of a ventricular septal defect, although the murmur of a small patent ductus is not coarse.
2. A patent ductus murmur has systolic and diastolic components, whereas a ventricular septal defect murmur is systolic.
3. A bounding pulse and wide pulse pressure are found in a child with patent ductus but not in a child with ventricular septal defect.
4. The murmur of patent ductus is loudest over the first and second intercostal spaces to the left of the sternal border. The murmur of ventricular septal defect is loudest in the third and fourth intercostal spaces.
5. In a large ventricular septal defect associated with a patent ductus arteriosus, there may be relatively little or no flow through the patent ductus arteriosus and thus no distinct murmur. As a result, the patent ductus may not be recognized. In a small ventricular septal defect, there may be a lower pulmonary artery pressure, and thus a greater blood flow through the patent ductus. Therefore, patent ductus arteriosus is more easily recognized in children with a small ventricular septal defect than in children with a large ventricular

septal defect.

Innocent Systolic Murmur

There is normally no problem differentiating a ventricular septal defect, generating a harsh holosystolic murmur, from an innocent systolic murmur, which is soft and diamond shaped (crescendo-decrescendo). If a distinction cannot be made on this basis, the following points may help to differentiate the two:

1. The innocent systolic murmur has a vibratory quality, whereas the murmur of ventricular septal defect is harsh.
2. The murmur of ventricular septal defect is localized in the third and fourth intercostal spaces to the left of the sternum. The innocent systolic murmur is usually not localized.
3. An innocent systolic murmur is widely transmitted to the aortic area and the neck, whereas the murmur of ventricular septal defect— although usually of greater intensity—is not as widely transmitted.
4. The murmur of ventricular septal defect obscures the first heart sound, whereas an innocent systolic murmur does not.
5. In a young infant whose pulmonary vascular resistance has not yet fallen, the murmur of a ventricular septal defect may not be holosystolic or characteristically harsh and may therefore be harder to distinguish from an innocent murmur.

Pulmonic Stenosis

Several points distinguish the murmur of ventricular septal defect from that of pulmonic stenosis. One of the most recognizable is that the murmur of pulmonic stenosis is very well transmitted to the lung fields, whereas the murmur of ventricular septal defect is not. Additional points include the following:

1. The murmur of ventricular septal defect is less coarse than the murmur of pulmonic stenosis.
2. The murmur of ventricular septal defect is loudest in the third or fourth intercostal spaces to the left of the sternum. The murmur of pulmonic stenosis is loudest at a higher point, around the second left intercostal space. If the ventricular septal defect is high, or the pulmonic stenosis is infundibular, the murmurs may be in the same place.
3. The murmur of ventricular septal defect is holosystolic, whereas the murmur of pulmonic stenosis is diamond shaped (crescendo-decrescendo).
4. The murmur of pulmonic stenosis may be associated with an ejection sound, whereas the murmur of ventricular septal defect is not. However, if there is an aneurysm of the ventricular septum, a

click is sometimes audible.

5. A ventricular septal defect may be associated with pulmonic stenosis, and both murmurs may be present, as in mild tetralogy of Fallot.

Mitral Regurgitation

Differentiating between the murmur of ventricular septal defect and that of mitral regurgitation is often difficult. Occasionally mitral insufficiency occurs together with a ventricular septal defect, and this must be borne in mind when making a distinction. Differentiating points include the following:

1. The murmur of ventricular septal defect is loudest over the left sternal border, but the murmur of mitral regurgitation is loudest over the apex and radiates into the left axilla.
2. The murmur of mitral regurgitation is usually less harsh than the murmur of ventricular septal defect, the former having a high-pitched blowing quality.

Other Differential Diagnoses

Aortic stenosis, especially subvalvular aortic stenosis, is a murmur that can be confused with ventricular septal defect, even by an experienced clinician. Atrial septal defect, especially atrial septal defect plus ventricular septal defect, can also be confused with the murmur of pure ventricular septal defect.

Prognosis

After surgical closure, a ventricular septal defect may be considered cured— if there is no residual murmur or right bundle branch block.

MITRAL REGURGITATION

Origin and Nature of the Murmur of Mitral Regurgitation

The murmur of mitral regurgitation (insufficiency) is generated by blood flowing through the mitral valve during systole, when it should be closed. The murmur is usually audible throughout systole (Figure 11-11), although if the mitral insufficiency is mild, the murmur may be loudest in early systole and not extend to the end of systole. The murmur is loudest over the apex, and because the murmur is high-pitched, it is best heard with the diaphragm of the stethoscope. If very loud, a mitral regurgitant murmur is transmitted to the left axilla.

In severe mitral insufficiency, increased forward blood flow may produce a murmur of relative mitral stenosis. If the valve ring is significantly dilated, the mitral stenosis murmur may not be heard. If the murmur is audible, the insufficiency is at least moderately severe. A loud third heart

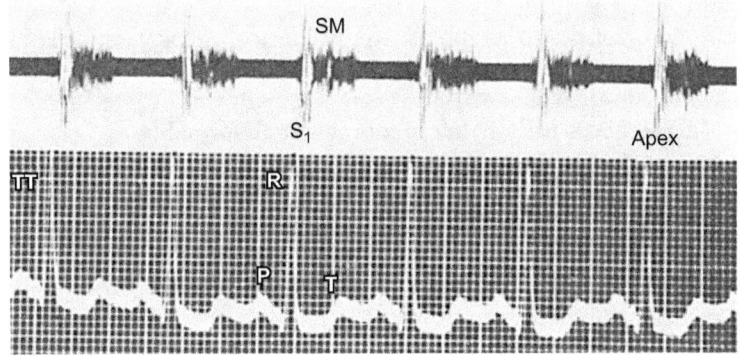

Figure 11-11. Holosystolic murmur of chronic mitral regurgitation. **SM**, Systolic murmur. (From Levine SA, Harvey WP: **Clinical auscultation of the heart,** ed 2, Philadelphia, 1959, WB Saunders.)

sound may also be heard in severe mitral insufficiency.

Causes of Mitral Regurgitation and Insufficiency

Mitral insufficiency in older children is associated with acquired rheumatic heart disease as well as with a number of congenital heart defects. In children of all ages, mitral insufficiency may, as in adults, occur secondary to left ventricular dilatation with severe ventricular dysfunction.

Rheumatic Heart Disease
Mitral insufficiency is most commonly caused by acute rheumatic fever. Sometimes there is no history of rheumatic fever, and the mitral insufficiency appears as an isolated finding.

Congenital Heart Defects
Endocardial Cushion Defects. Infants with complete common atrioventricular (AV) canal often experience congestive heart failure and become dusky or cyanotic when they cry, feed, or strain. These defects are common in children with Down syndrome (see Chapter 3). Affected children have both atrial and ventricular defects and may also have mitral or tricuspid regurgitation. Children with milder AV canal defects, such as ostium primum atrial septal defect, may have a competently functioning mitral valve, but the valve is almost always displaced, and there is a cleft in the anterior valve leaflet. Insufficiency may appear only after repair of the atrial septal defect (see Figure 15-6).

Corrected Transposition of the Great Arteries. In corrected transposition of the great arteries (see Figure 15-13), the AV valve on the left side is really the tricuspid valve because ventricular inversion is present. There is a relatively high incidence of Ebstein's anomaly (see Chapter 15) and insufficiency of this left-sided valve.

Isolated Congenital Mitral Insufficiency. In isolated congenital mitral insufficiency, the child may have concomitant patent ductus arteriosus, a ventricular septal defect, or a small atrial septal defect, but mitral insufficiency is usually the predominant abnormality.

Congenital Mitral Insufficiency Associated With Coarctation of the Aorta. In congenital mitral insufficiency, the coarctation increases the severity of the mitral regurgitation. After surgical correction of the coarctation, the degree of regurgitation usually diminishes.

Anomalous Left Coronary Artery. If the left coronary artery originates from the pulmonary artery, it causes ischemic damage to the left ventricle and papillary muscle (Figure 11-12). Typically the patient is an infant with an enlarged heart, mitral regurgitation, and distinctive findings

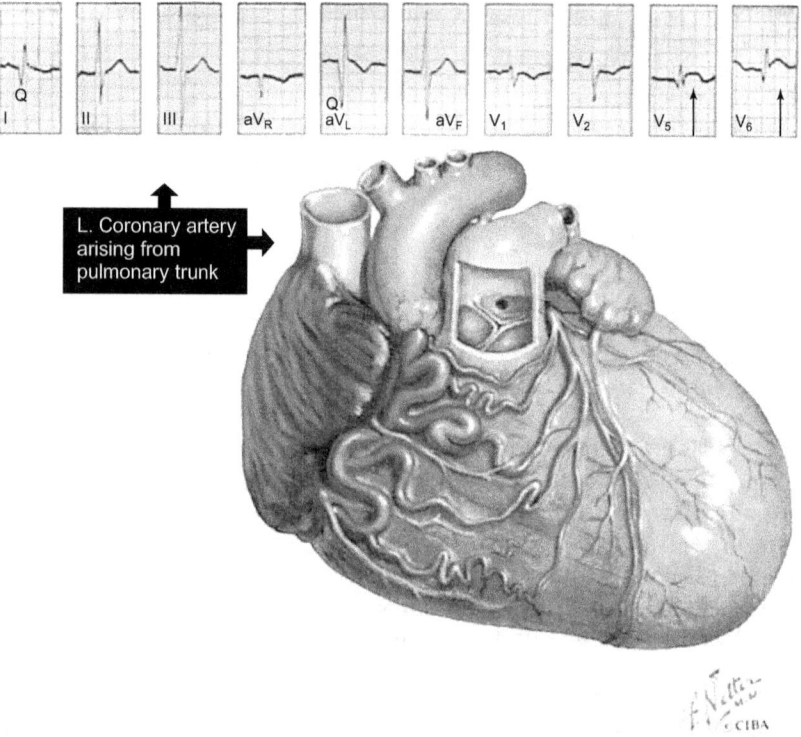

Figure 11-12. Anomalous left coronary artery arising from pulmonary trunk. Note that the normal right coronary artery and its branches have become dilated and tortuous, whereas the left coronary artery remains small. The ECG has abnormal Q waves in leads I and AVL, as well as ST segment elevation in leads V_5 and V_6 **(arrows)**, indicating myocardial ischemia. (Modified from Van Mierop LH: Diseases—congenital anomalies. In Yonkman F, editor: **Heart,** Summit, NJ, 1969, Ciba-Geigy.)

on the electrocardiogram (abnormal Q waves in leads I and AVL and evidence of left ventricular ischemia). The definitive diagnosis is made with an angiogram that visualizes the aortic root and coronary arteries. One must keep in mind that any lesion causing poor myocardial function, especially of the left ventricle, can, as a result of left ventricular dilatation, give rise to mitral insufficiency.

Mitral Leaflet Prolapse. In 17% of cases, the midsystolic click (or clicks) of mitral leaflet prolapse (see Chapter 9) is followed by a late systolic murmur, the **click-murmur syndrome** (Figure 11-13). When the murmur is soft, it does not radiate widely from the apex and is often missed or misinterpreted as innocent. Mild exercise and having the patient lie on the left side during auscultation bring out the murmur. It reaches a crescendo late in systole and may be musical, a "lub-shoo-OP" sound. In some children, the murmur is a loud whoop or honk that may be audible several centimeters from the chest and can startle the parents.

In more severe cases of mitral leaflet prolapse, the murmur is holo-

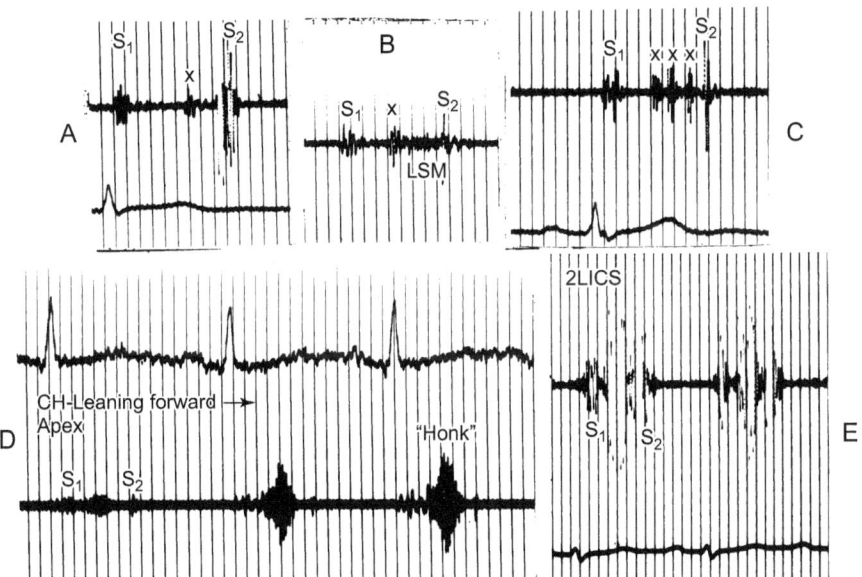

Figure 11-13. Mitral leaflet prolapse. **A**, Isolated late systolic click **(X)**. **B**, Midsystolic click and late systolic murmur **(LSM)**. **C**, Multiple clicks in midsystole to late systole. **D**, The evolution of a systolic honk as the patient leans forward in held expiration. **E**, Multiple clicks interrupting a long systolic murmur recorded at the base. Eight hours later, this and any other murmur was absent. **2LIS**, Second left intercostal space. (From Gingell RL, Vlad P: Mitral valve prolapse. In Keith JD, Rowe RD, Vlad P, editors: **Heart disease in infancy and childhood,** ed 3, New York, 1978, Macmillan.)

systolic. Because of its long duration, this murmur is rarely mistaken for an innocent murmur.

TRICUSPID REGURGITATION

Origin and Nature of the Murmur of Tricuspid Regurgitation

The murmur of tricuspid regurgitation (insufficiency) begins with the first heart sound. When faint, the murmur is short and decrescendo. When loud, it is holosystolic and may radiate as far as the left anterior axillary line. The murmur is best heard to the left of the lower end of the sternum—in contrast to the murmur of mitral insufficiency, which is loudest over the apex. Characteristically, this murmur is louder during inspiration—in contrast to the murmur of mitral insufficiency, which is unaffected by respiration (Figure 11-14).

Causes of Tricuspid Regurgitation

A number of disorders may cause tricuspid regurgitation in children. These include **Ebstein's anomaly** (see Chapter 15), large ventricular septal defects accompanied by pulmonary hypertension, dilatation of the right ventricle and tricuspid annulus (now relatively uncommon), **rheumatic valvular disease,** and **atrioventricular canal defects,** especially after cardiac surgery when the remaining tissue is scanty, most having been used to fix an incompetent mitral valve. Surgical repairs of complete transposition of the great arteries using atrial tissue to construct the interatrial baffle (**Mustard** or **Senning operation**) may also cause tricuspid insufficiency (Figure 11-15). In these cases, the right ventricle is the systemic ventricle. Tricuspid insufficiency may also result from surgical correction of tetralogy of Fallot, if right ventricular function is poor and pulmonary insufficiency is a problem. Generally, the murmur of tricuspid regurgitation is not heard unless right ventricular pressure is elevated.

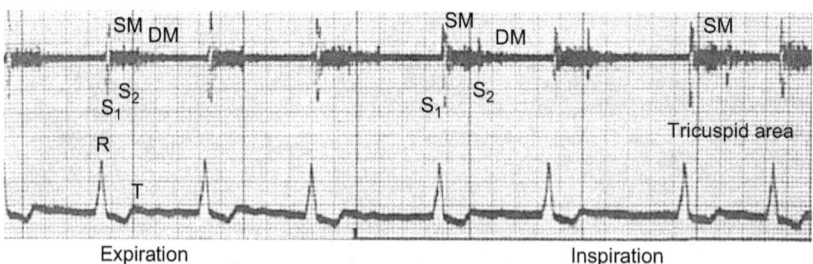

Figure 11-14. Holosystolic murmur of tricuspid regurgitation with inspiratory augmentation of murmur. **DM,** Diastolic murmur; **SM,** systolic murmur. (From Levine SA, Harvey WP: **Clinical auscultation of the heart,** ed 2, Philadelphia, 1959, WB Saunders.)

VALVULAR AORTIC STENOSIS
Origin of the Murmur of Aortic Stenosis

Valvular aortic stenosis is the most common cause of left ventricular obstruction in children and adults. The stenosis may be present at birth, or

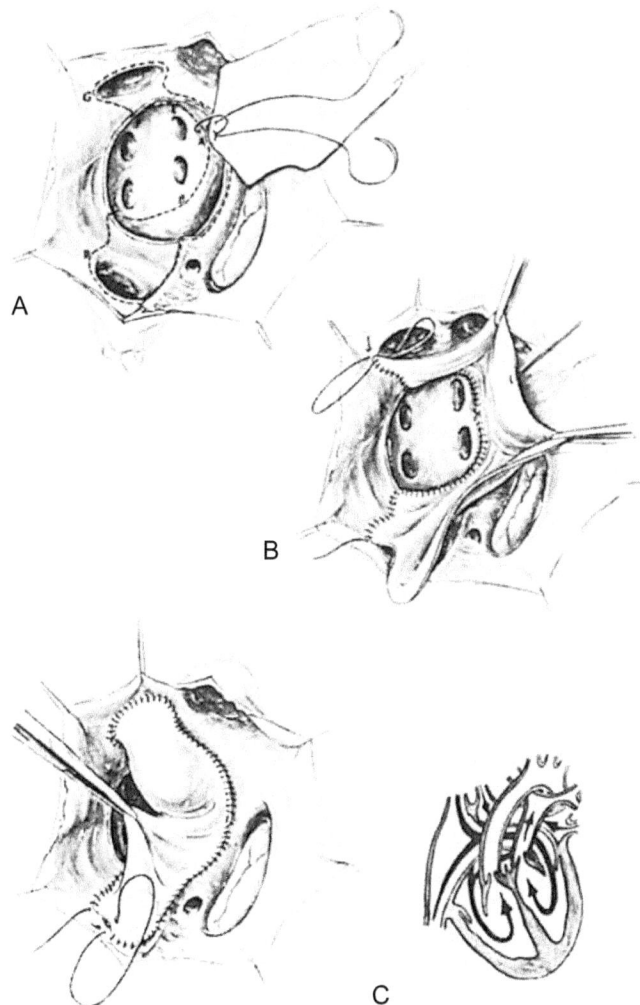

Figure 11-15. The Mustard operation, with interatrial baffle to invert venous return to correct transposition of the great arteries. **A** to **C**, The patch is sutured into place to divert systemic venous return to the mitral valve. Pulmonary and coronary venous blood pass to the tricuspid valve. (From Barratt-Boyes BG: **Heart disease in infancy: diagnosis and surgical treatment,** Edinburgh, 1973, Churchill Livingstone.)

it may develop gradually because of fibrosis and calcification of a congenitally malformed valve. Rheumatic aortic stenosis is extremely uncommon in children and is usually associated with significant aortic regurgitation. Aortic stenosis in children is often associated with a bicuspid aortic valve, which may predispose to development of aortic aneurysm later in life.

Nature of the Murmur of Aortic Stenosis

The murmur of aortic stenosis is crescendo-decrescendo. It builds up to a peak in midsystole and then diminishes in loudness. When recorded on a phonocardiogram, the murmur has a diamond shape (Figure 11-16).

The murmur of aortic stenosis is loudest in the first and second right intercostal spaces and has a harsh, rough quality, like the sound made by clearing the throat. The murmur is transmitted well to the neck, especially to the right side. In infants and children under 5 years of age, the murmur may be loudest at the left sternal border and toward the apex. As the stenosis becomes more severe, the murmur becomes louder and longer and peaks later. Children with loud murmurs usually have more severe stenosis than children with soft murmurs.

In almost all infants and children with valvular aortic stenosis, the murmur is preceded by an ejection click, generated by the sudden arrest of

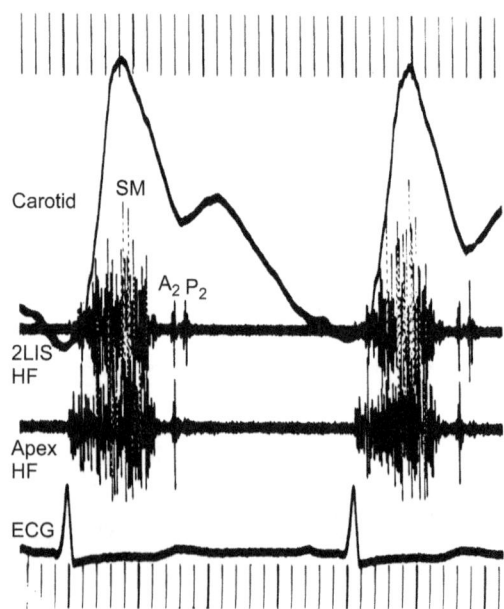

Figure 11-16. Loud diamond-shaped murmur of aortic stenosis. Note that the peak intensity of the murmur occurs well before the second sound. **2LIS,** Second left intercostal space; **HF,** high frequency; **SM,** systolic murmur. (From Nadas AS, Fyler DC: **Pediatric cardiology,** ed 3, Philadelphia, WB Saunders, 1972. Copyright AS Nadas.)

the domed stenotic valve when it has opened to its limit. The click is loudest at the apex and left sternal border, and it does not vary with respiration.

If the stenosis is subvalvular (in the aortic ring), the click is absent. Thus, the presence or absence of the click helps to differentiate between valvular and subvalvular stenosis (Figure 11-17). Subvalvular aortic stenosis is also commonly associated with aortic insufficiency.

Differentiating Aortic Stenosis From Other Conditions

Pulmonic Stenosis

The murmurs of aortic and pulmonic stenosis often can be differentiated by their locations and where they produce palpable thrills. The murmur of aortic stenosis is loudest in the aortic area, whereas the murmur of pulmonic stenosis is loudest in the pulmonic area. The thrill in a child with a loud (grades IV to VI) murmur of aortic stenosis is palpable on the right side of the neck, toward the shoulder. The thrill of pulmonic stenosis, in contrast, is palpable toward the left side of the neck and shoulder. The murmur of aortic stenosis is transmitted very well to the right carotid, whereas the murmur of pulmonic stenosis radiates to the lung fields. Both murmurs are palpable in

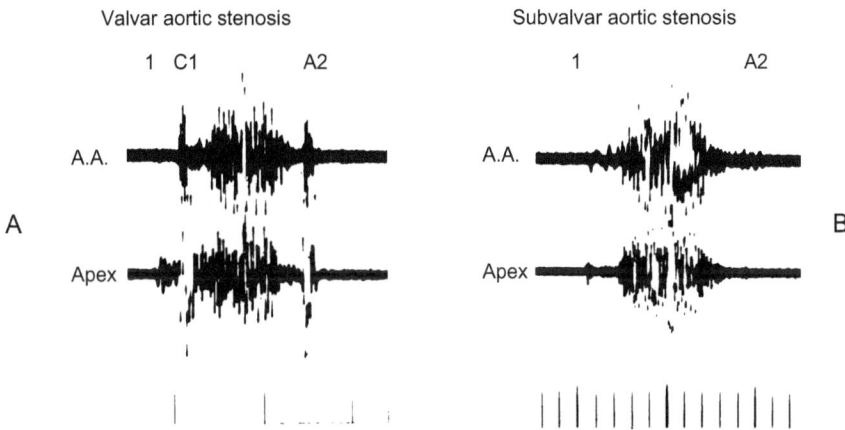

Figure 11-17. A comparison of the sounds and murmurs in aortic valvular stenosis and subvalvular aortic ring stenosis. A, The tracing of aortic valve stenosis shows a relatively faint first heart sound, a well-heard systolic click, an ejection-type systolic murmur, and a clearly demonstrable aortic second sound. B, On the other hand, with subvalvular aortic stenosis, although the first sound was faint, there was no audible systolic click, and the aortic valve closure showed minimal vibrations at both the aortic area and the apex, which would obviously be inaudible with the stethoscope. These findings are often helpful in differentiating between the two types of aortic stenosis. **A.A.,** Aortic area. (From Olley PM, Bloom KR, Rowe RD: Aortic stenosis: valvular, subaortic, and supravalvular. In Keith JD, Rowe RD, Vlad P, editors: **Heart disease in infancy and childhood,** ed 3, New York, 1978, Macmillan. Courtesy Dr. CM Oakley, Postgraduate Medical School, Hammersmith, London, England.)

the suprasternal notch.

Innocent Murmur

The murmur of valvular aortic stenosis is accompanied by an ejection sound, whereas an innocent murmur is not. It is also usually harsher than an innocent murmur.

Ventricular Septal Defect

The murmur of aortic stenosis is coarser than the murmur of ventricular septal defect and is associated with an ejection click. In addition, the murmur of ventricular septal defect is usually holosystolic and is heard best at the lower left sternal border, rather than higher on the precordium.

Mitral Insufficiency

Differentiating mitral insufficiency from aortic stenosis is not usually a diagnostic problem. If confusion exists, the two murmurs may be most easily differentiated by where they are heard. The murmur of aortic stenosis is transmitted well to the apex, whereas the murmur of mitral insufficiency is poorly transmitted to the aortic area. Therefore, if a murmur sounds the same in the two areas, it is probably caused by aortic stenosis.

MUSCULAR SUBAORTIC STENOSIS

Origin of the Murmur of Muscular Subaortic Stenosis

Muscular subaortic stenosis, also called **idiopathic hypertrophic subaortic stenosis** (IHSS) or **hypertrophic obstructive cardiomyopathy,** is genetic and is transmitted as an autosomal dominant trait. In some patients, the characteristic murmur is evident only if the left ventricle is stressed by hypertension or aortic valvular stenosis. Muscular subaortic stenosis may sometimes be associated with other cardiac abnormalities, such as atrial septal defect, endocardial cushion defects, or pulmonic stenosis. It occurs equally often in girls and boys but is rarely found in Africans or black Americans. Although muscular subaortic stenosis has been found in all age groups, from newborns onward, patients usually do not begin to develop symptoms until after 30 years of age.

Nature of the Murmur of Muscular Subaortic Stenosis

Certain characteristics are typical of the murmur of muscular subaortic stenosis and may help to differentiate it from other murmurs. The murmur is poorly transmitted to the second right intercostal space and, rarely, to the neck. It ends before the second heart sound but is not always diamond shaped. The aortic second sound is normal and well heard at the apex. Third and fourth heart sounds may also be present. Aortic ejection clicks are very rare.

The Valsalva maneuver may help to emphasize the murmur of

muscular subaortic stenosis. While the patient strains, the murmur becomes louder and harsher. The murmur is also profoundly affected by changes in patient position. Squatting quickly diminishes the murmur, whereas standing suddenly accentuates it and possibly the fourth heart sound as well.

Differentiating Subaortic Stenosis From Other Conditions

Aortic Stenosis

In contrast to the murmur of subaortic stenosis, the murmur of aortic valvular stenosis is transmitted well to the second right intercostal space and the neck. The murmur is usually diamond shaped and is either unaffected by the Valsalva maneuver or made softer. It is also often accompanied by a click.

Ventricular Septal Defect

It may be difficult to differentiate subaortic stenosis from ventricular septal defect; the Valsalva maneuver, if the child can perform it, can be helpful in making the distinction. In contrast to the murmur of subaortic stenosis, the murmur of ventricular septal defect tends to be eliminated by the Valsalva maneuver.

Discrete Fibrous Subaortic Stenosis

Discrete fibrous subaortic stenosis is different from idiopathic muscular subaortic stenosis. The murmur of discrete fibrous subaortic stenosis is loudest at the middle left sternal border, may have a honking quality, and is often associated with mild aortic insufficiency. Discrete fibrous subaortic stenosis presents a difficult diagnostic challenge but can be distinguished from ventricular septal defect or valvular aortic stenosis by echocardiography.

SUPRAVALVULAR AORTIC STENOSIS

Origin of the Murmur of Supravalvular Aortic Stenosis

Supravalvular aortic stenosis is a narrowing of the ascending aorta just above the sinuses of Valsalva (Figure 11-18). There are two main types of supravalvular aortic stenosis: (1) an hourglass narrowing of the aorta, occurring in two thirds of the cases, and (2) a diffuse narrowing of the aortic lumen. Supravalvular aortic stenosis may be one of multiple cardiac abnormalities, and some affected children have Williams syndrome,[*] with a characteristic elfin face (Figure 11-19), mild mental retardation, and other heart abnormalities (Figure 11-20).

Genetics

Supravalvular aortic stenosis is inherited as an autosomal dominant charac-

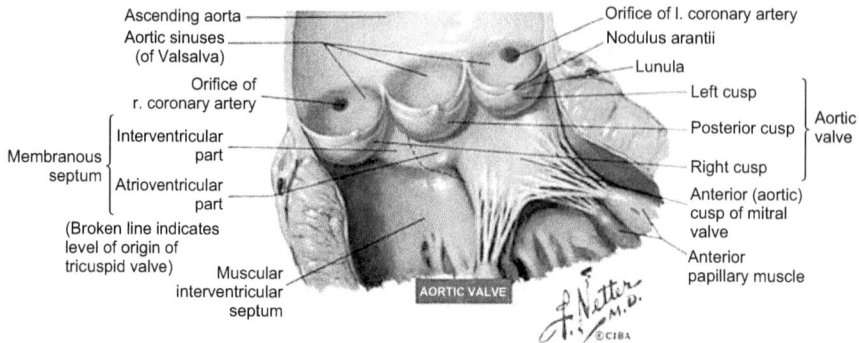

Figure 11-18. Section through the aortic valve, showing the sinuses of Valsalva. The coronary arteries open into these sinuses. In patients with supravalvular aortic stenosis, the aortic narrowing begins just above the sinuses of Valsalva. (From Van Mierop LH: Diseases— congenital anomalies. In Yonkman F, editor: **Heart,** Summit, NJ, 1969, Ciba-Geigy.)

teristic. The defect is in the elastin gene, chromosome 7q11.23, and causes reduced elastin content during development. Williams syndrome is sporadic and is also due to a 7q11.23 defect of elastin and adjacent genes.

Nature of the Murmur of Supravalvular Aortic Stenosis

Supravalvular aortic stenosis causes an ejection systolic murmur. This murmur is maximal in the aortic area and is conducted well to the carotid arteries. The murmur is loud, grades IV to VI, and is usually discovered before the child is 1 year old. A thrill is invariably palpable in the suprasternal notch, and the aortic second sound is accentuated. The arterial pulse is more prominent in the right arm and the systolic pressure is higher there, the result of a high-velocity jet of blood directed into the innominate artery.

Ross Procedure

Some surgeons now perform the Ross procedure in children with severely

---

* Classified as a nonverbal learning disability, Williams syndrome is associated with speech and language aptitude that far exceeds other cognitive abilities. One patient with Williams syndrome, for example, could scribble only a few clumsy lines when asked to draw an elephant but could describe the animal in exquisite detail: "It has long gray ears, fan ears, ears that can blow in the wind. It has a long trunk that can pick up grass or pick up hay." The most striking cognitive aspect of Williams syndrome is an affinity and talent for music. Many people with Williams syndrome have perfect pitch, the ability to identify any musical note they hear. They also have an uncanny rhythmic ability. One boy with Williams syndrome was taught to tap a complex 7/4 time rhythm with one hand while keeping 4/4 time with the other. A child with Williams syndrome has a short attention span for many tasks but can spend hours listening to or making music. The opera singer Gloria Lenhoff, a 46-year-old lyric soprano with perfect pitch and Williams syndrome, can sing 2500 songs in 25 languages, flawlessly accented. However, because her IQ is 55, Ms. Lenhoff cannot subtract three from five or make change for a dollar. (From Maher, BA: Music, the brain, and Williams syndrome, **The Scientist,** Nov 26, 2001, pp 20-21.)

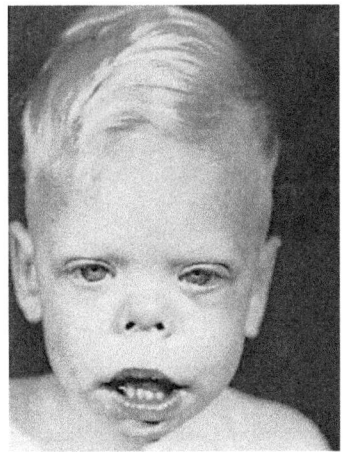
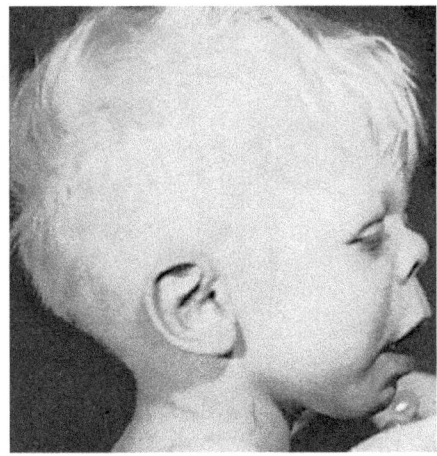

Figure 11-19. Williams syndrome. Note the small mandible, large maxilla, and upturned nose. (From Nadas AS, Fyler DC: **Pediatric cardiology,** ed 3, Philadelphia, 1972, WB Saunders. Copyright AS Nadas.)

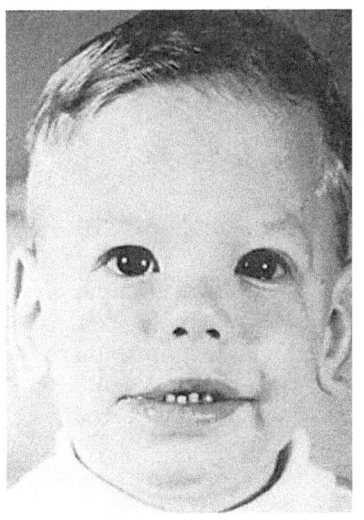

Figure 11-20. Williams syndrome. Facial appearance of a boy with bilateral stenosis of the pulmonary arteries, supravalvular aortic stenosis, mental retardation, and infantile hypercalcemia. The chin is small, the mouth large, the lips patulous, the nose blunt and upturned, the eyes wideset, the forehead broad, the cheeks baggy, and the teeth malformed. (From Perloff JK: **Physical examination of the heart and circulation,** ed 3, Philadelphia, 2000, WB Saunders.)

diseased aortic valves. The patient's pulmonic valve is placed in the aortic position, and a homograft in the pulmonary position (Figure 11-21). This approach is a response to the difficulty of adequately repairing severely stenosed aortic valves in children without inducing aortic insufficiency and the problems associated with use of prosthetic valves in children (see Chapter 14). Cardiologists hope that the Ross valves will grow along with the patients and will prove long-lasting.

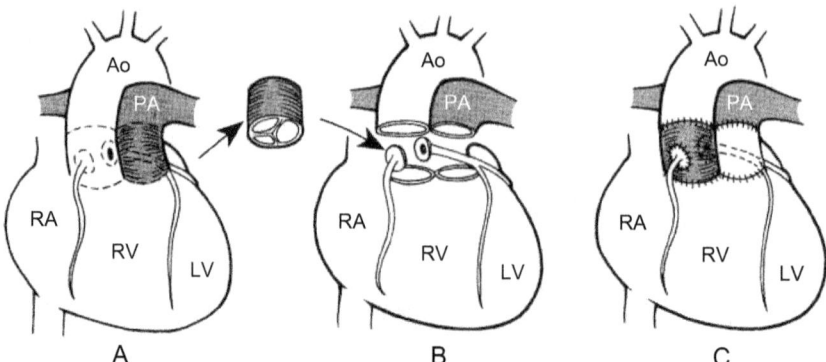

Figure 11-21. Ross procedure (pulmonary root autograft). **A,** Two horizontal lines on the aorta and pulmonary artery **(PA)** and two broken circles around the coronary artery ostia are lines of proposed incision. The pulmonic valve with a small rim of right ventricular **(RV)** muscle and the adjacent PA are removed. **B,** The aortic valve and the adjacent aorta have been removed, leaving buttons of aortic tissue around the coronary arteries. **C,** The pulmonary autograft is sutured to the aortic annulus and to the distal aorta, and the coronary arteries are sutured to openings made in the pulmonary artery. The pulmonic valve is replaced with either an aortic or pulmonary allograft. **Ao,** Aorta; **LV,** left ventricle; **RA,** right atrium. (From Park MK: **Pediatric cardiology for practitioners,** ed 3, St Louis, 1996, Mosby.)

PULMONIC STENOSIS

Origin of the Murmur of Pulmonic Stenosis

Stenosis of the pulmonic valve or pulmonary artery is often present from birth (Figure 11-22). Most commonly, there is a stenosed valve, which is dome-shaped with a narrow outlet (Figure 11-23). Children with the most severe pulmonic stenosis, **critical pulmonic stenosis,** may also have abnormal ventricles, may be blue as neonates, and may require shunts and valvulotomy (a surgical incision that frees up the valve leaflets). These children often have a chubby, round, "moonface" and healthy appearance (Figure 11-24).

In a few cases of pulmonic stenosis, the valve is dysplastic (abnormally developed) because of thickening of all three leaflets, which remain discrete and separated. These children have a distinct facial appearance with a small jaw, wide-set eyes, low-set ears, and drooping eyelids (Figure 11-25). This condition, called **Noonan syndrome,** is associated with a normal chromosome complement. Affected children, some of whom are boys, have other stigmata of **Turner syndrome** (Figure 11-26), which is found in girls with a single X chromosome.

A third group of children with supravalvular stenosis of the pulmonary artery have Williams syndrome. These children have a characteristic facial appearance, mild mental retardation, and other heart abnormalities (see Figure 11-19). In other cases, maternal rubella may be the cause of peripheral

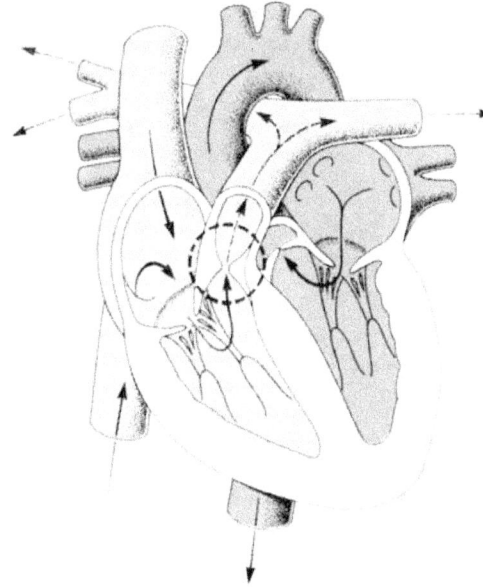

Figure 11-22. Pulmonic stenosis (valvar). Blood flow through the pulmonary artery is diminished, as illustrated by the broken arrows. (From Foster R, Hunsberger MM, Anderson JT: **Family-centered nursing care of children,** Philadelphia, 1990, WB Saunders.)

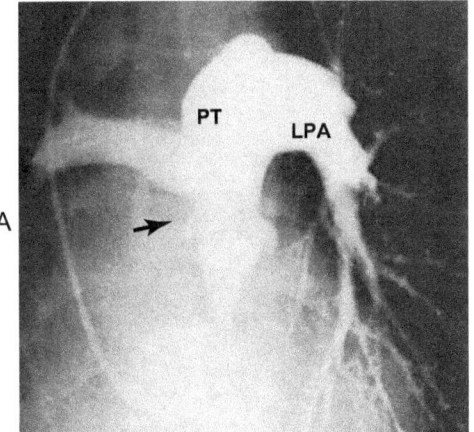

A

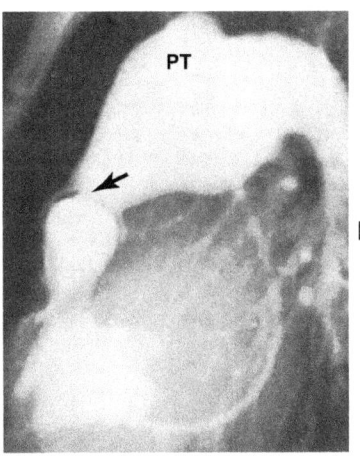

B

Figure 11-23. A and B, Angiocardiogram with contrast material injected into the right ventricle of a 47-year-old woman with severe pulmonic valvar stenosis (gradient of 106 mm Hg). A, In the posteroanterior projection, dilatation of the pulmonary trunk (PT) is not evident, but the left branch (LPA) is conspicuously dilated. Arrow points to the level of the stenotic valve. B, In the lateral projection, the dome-shaped stenotic pulmonic valve (arrow) is easily seen, and poststenotic dilatation of the pulmonary trunk is readily apparent. (From Perloff JK: **The clinical recognition of congenital heart disease,** ed 4, Philadelphia, 1994, WB Saunders.)

Continued

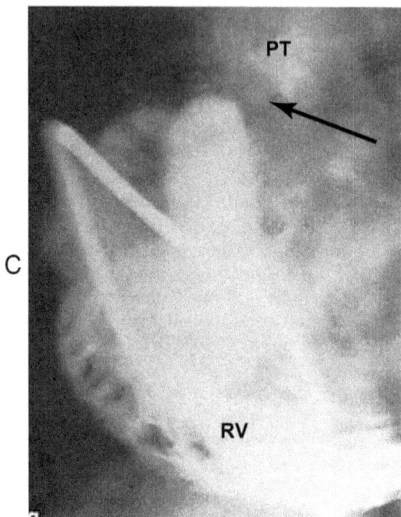
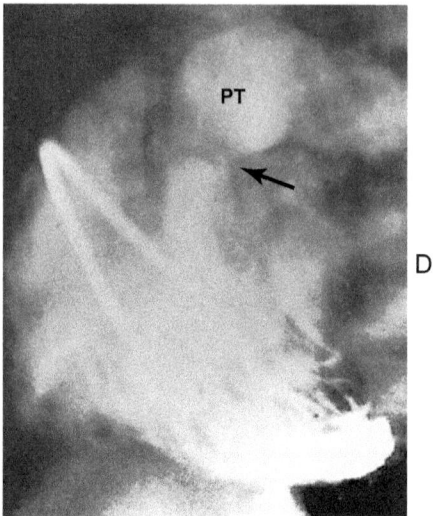

C

D

Figure 11-23, cont'd. C and D, Angiocardiogram (left anterior oblique projection) with contrast material injected into the right ventricle **(RV)** of a 10-month-old girl with severe pulmonic valve stenosis (right ventricular pressure exceeds systemic pressure). **C,** The right ventricle **(RV)** and infundibulum are filled, and a wisp of dye enters the pulmonary trunk. **D,** The dome-shaped stenotic valve **(arrow)** is easily seen, together with poststenotic dilatation of the pulmonary trunk **(PT).** (From Perloff JK: **The clinical recognition of congenital heart disease,** ed 4, Philadelphia, 1994, WB Saunders.)

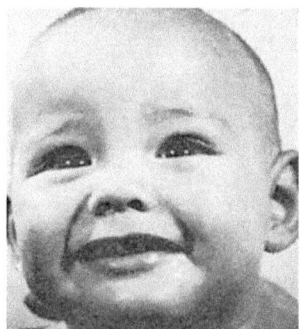

Figure 11-24. The chubby, round face and healthy appearance of an infant with isolated valvular pulmonic stenosis. (From Perloff JK: **Physical examination of the heart and circulation,** ed 3, Philadelphia, 2000, WB Saunders.)

pulmonary arterial stenosis.

Nature of the Murmur of Pulmonic Stenosis

Thrill

The murmur of pulmonic stenosis is often accompanied by a thrill that corresponds with the location and intensity of the murmur. When the

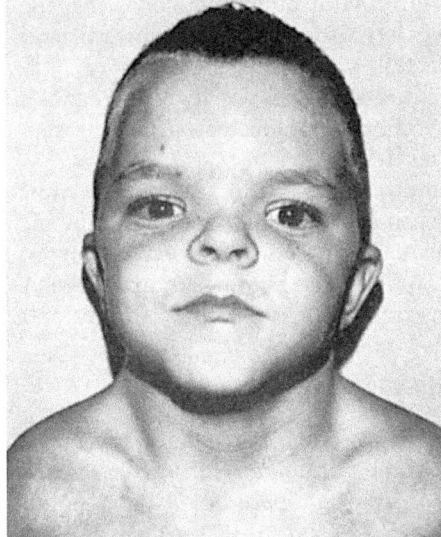

Figure 11-25. A boy with Noonan syndrome and pulmonary arterial stenosis. (From Rowe RD: Supravalvular aortic stenosis. In Keith J, Rowe R, Vlad P, editors: **Heart disease in infancy and childhood,** ed 3, New York, 1978, Macmillan.)

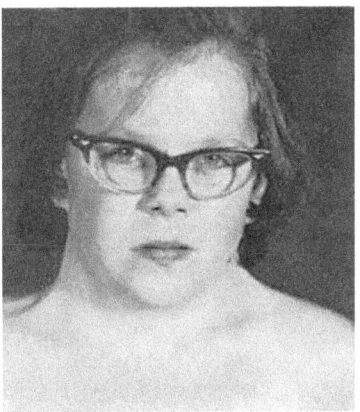
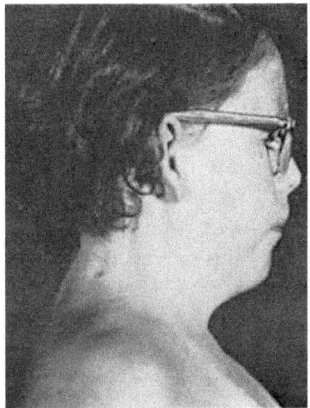

Figure 11-26. Turner syndrome. Note webbing of the neck. Coarctation of the aorta occurs frequently in patients with Turner syndrome. (From Nadas AS, Fyler DC: **Pediatric cardiology,** ed 3, Philadelphia, 1972, WB Saunders. Copyright AS Nadas.)

pulmonic valve is stenotic, the thrill is greatest in the second or third left intercostal space. The thrill may radiate upward and to the left because the jet from the valve is directed to the left pulmonary artery. The thrill may also be felt in the suprasternal notch. In addition, a strong right ventricular systolic impulse at the lower left sternal border may occur.

Heart Sounds

The first heart sound is normal in children with pulmonic stenosis. If the stenotic valve is dome-shaped, an **ejection sound** closely follows S_1 and must be distinguished from it. The ejection sound is loudest during expiration and diminishes on inspiration (Figure 11-27). As the degree of stenosis increases, the separation of S_1 and the ejection sound decreases, the duration of the murmur increases, and the peak is delayed.

In cases of severe stenosis, the ejection click is absent, the long murmur obscures the aortic component of the second heart sound, and the pulmonic component is greatly diminished or absent. There is also increased splitting of the aortic and pulmonic components as the stenosis becomes more severe. A fourth heart sound may develop from right ventricular hypertrophy and decreasing right ventricular compliance.

Postoperative Murmur

After surgical correction of pulmonic stenosis, there may be a grade I or II systolic murmur caused by turbulence in the pulmonary outflow tract. This murmur is in the second or third left intercostal space but is shorter and softer than the preoperative murmur.

Differentiating the Murmurs of Pulmonic Stenosis

The ejection sound is valuable in distinguishing mobile dome-type pulmonic stenosis from dysplastic stenosis, discrete subvalvular obstruction, and stenosis of the pulmonary artery branches. Only the mobile dome-type stenosis has an ejection sound; dysplastic stenosis, discrete subvalvular obstruction, and stenosis of the pulmonary artery branches do not. In very severe pulmonic stenosis (as in aortic stenosis), the ejection sound may disappear as the narrowing increases.

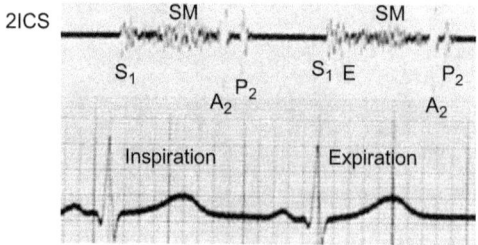

Figure 11-27. Phonocardiograms from a 9-year-old girl with mild pulmonic valve stenosis (gradient of 25 mm Hg). In the second left intercostal space **(2ICS),** a pulmonic ejection sound **(E)** is absent during inspiration and present during expiration. A midsystolic murmur **(SM)** just reaches the aortic component of the second heart sound **(A_2).** The pulmonic component **(P_2)** is clearly evident and only slightly delayed. The split second heart sound widens on inspiration and narrows but persists on expiration. (From Perloff JK: **The clinical recognition of congenital heart disease,** ed 4, Philadelphia, 1994, WB Saunders.)

Prognosis

Many children do well after surgical correction of pulmonic stenosis, although they may be left with some residual pulmonary insufficiency.

DILATATION OF THE PULMONARY ARTERY NEAR THE PULMONIC VALVE

Some cases of dilatation of the pulmonary artery are of unknown cause and are found in otherwise normal children. Other cases are associated with pulmonary hypertension, and many are the result of congenital heart defects.

Origin and Nature of the Murmur of Pulmonary Dilatation

The murmur of pulmonary dilatation is generated by the ejection of blood into the dilated pulmonary trunk. The murmur is short, midsystolic, and loudest in the second left intercostal space and is heard best during expiration with the diaphragm of the stethoscope.

Thrill

It may be possible to see and palpate a systolic impulse over the second left intercostal space, especially during held exhalation. A pulmonic ejection sound and a prominent pulmonic component of the second heart sound may be palpable as well.

Heart Sounds

A **pulmonic ejection sound** is a consistent finding in dilatation of the pulmonary artery of unknown cause. To hear the sound, the stethoscope should be placed over the second left intercostal space. The ejection sound is usually well separated from the first heart sound. It becomes louder with expiration and softer with inspiration (Figure 11-28).

In some cases, wide splitting of the second heart sound is detectable. Although the split is wide, it is not fixed, and it lengthens on inspiration.

ATRIAL SEPTAL DEFECT

Origin of the Murmur of Atrial Septal Defect

An atrial septal defect is a communication between the right and left atria that, in the absence of any other abnormalities, produces left to right shunting. The resultant murmur is generated by increased blood flow through the pulmonic valve.

Nature of the Murmur of Atrial Septal Defect

Figure 11-28. Phonocardiograms of a 16-year-old girl with idiopathic dilatation of the pulmonary artery from the second and fourth left intercostal spaces (**2ICS, 4ICS**) with carotid pulse (**CAR**) and electrocardiogram. The first heart sound (**S₁**) is followed by a prominent pulmonic ejection sound (**E**) that selectively decreases during inspiration. The second heart sound (**A₂**, aortic component; **P₂**, pulmonic component) remains split during expiration but widens appropriately during inspiration. A short midsystolic murmur (**SM**) is present. (From Perloff JK: **The clinical recognition of congenital heart disease,** ed 4, Philadelphia, 1994, WB Saunders.)

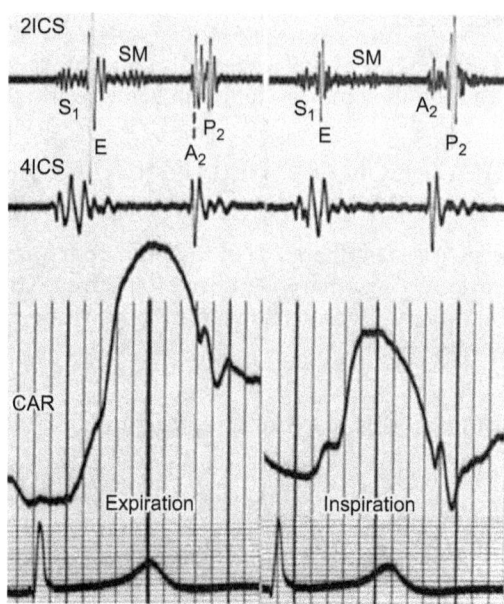

Even in its mildest forms, an atrial septal defect is associated with a systolic murmur and wide fixed splitting of the second heart sound (Figure 11-29). The murmur is soft, often less than grade III, and is crescendo-decrescendo, peaking in midsystole and ending well before the second heart sound. It is best heard with the stethoscope over the second left intercostal space. The wide, fixed splitting of the second sound allows differentiation between the murmur of an atrial septal defect and an innocent murmur in the same location. In an innocent murmur, the splitting of the second heart sound varies with respiration and is not wide and fixed. Nevertheless, differentiation between an innocent murmur and the murmur of atrial septal defect may be difficult.

In patients with a large atrial septal defect, a rumbling diastolic murmur may exist along the left border of the sternum or between the apex and the left border of the sternum. The murmur occurs because of increased blood flow through the tricuspid valve and consequently a relative tricuspid stenosis. In some patients, the tricuspid component of the first heart sound is increased at the apex or the left sternal edge.

Pulmonary hypertension is not a common complication of atrial septal defect in children, but it is seen in adults older than 30 years of age. When pulmonary hypertension is present, the pulmonary component of the second heart sound is louder than usual, whereas the systolic murmur is soft or absent.

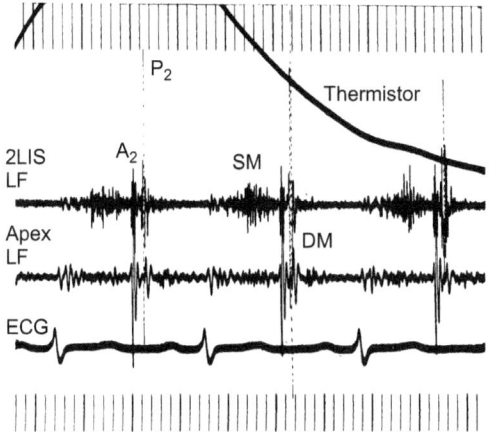

Figure 11-29. Low-intensity systolic ejection murmur in a patient with atrial septal defect. Note also the well-split second heart sound and the low-frequency early diastolic murmur **(DM).** The thermistor indicates the phase of respiration: inspiration **(left),** expiration **(right). 2LIS,** Second left intercostal space; **LF,** low frequency, **SM,** systolic murmur. (From Nadas AS, Fyler DC: **Pediatric cardiology,** ed 3, Philadelphia, 1972, WB Saunders. Copyright AS Nadas.)

Additional Physical Findings in Atrial Septal Defect

It may be possible to palpate a conspicuous right ventricular impulse, which is especially prominent along the left sternal border during held expiration and in the subxyphoid region during held inspiration. A dilated, pulsatile pulmonary trunk may also be palpable in the left second intercostal space.

Children with an atrial septal defect are occasionally underweight, small, frail, and slender. Retraction of the skin along the ribs (Harrison's grooves) indicates poor pulmonary compliance ("stiff lungs"). When an ostium secundum atrial septal defect is part of the Holt-Oram syndrome (a rare autosomal dominant syndrome), the child has an underdeveloped thumb with an extra phalanx, making apposition of the thumb and finger difficult, and giving the thumb a crooked appearance. In some cases, the thumb is rudimentary or completely absent. In others, the radius is under-developed, making it difficult to turn the hand palm up. Additional con-genital syndromes associated with atrial septal defect are listed in Table 3-2.

Differentiating Atrial Septal Defect From Other Conditions

Pulmonic Valvular Stenosis
It is sometimes difficult to tell the difference between an atrial septal defect and mild pulmonic valvular stenosis, because both produce a similar murmur and widely split second sounds. The following points may help to make this distinction:

1. In patients with pulmonic stenosis, the splitting of the second heart sound is likely to diminish during expiration, whereas in patients with atrial septal defect, the splitting is wide and fixed.

2. Usually, patients with pulmonic stenosis have a pulmonic ejection click, but in those with an atrial septal defect, a pulmonic ejection sound is not audible unless the patient also has pulmonary hypertension, an extremely unlikely event in children.
3. A patient with a large atrial septal defect often has a middiastolic tricuspid flow murmur, but a patient with pulmonic stenosis does not.

Prognosis

Patients may be considered cured after a successful surgical or transcatheter closure of a simple atrial septal defect (Figure 11-30).

COARCTATION OF THE AORTA
Origin of the Murmur of Coarctation of the Aorta

A common form of coarctation of the aorta is illustrated in Figure 11-31. Coarctation is suggested by the presence of upper extremity hypertension and pulses that are more forceful in the arms than in the legs. Moreover,

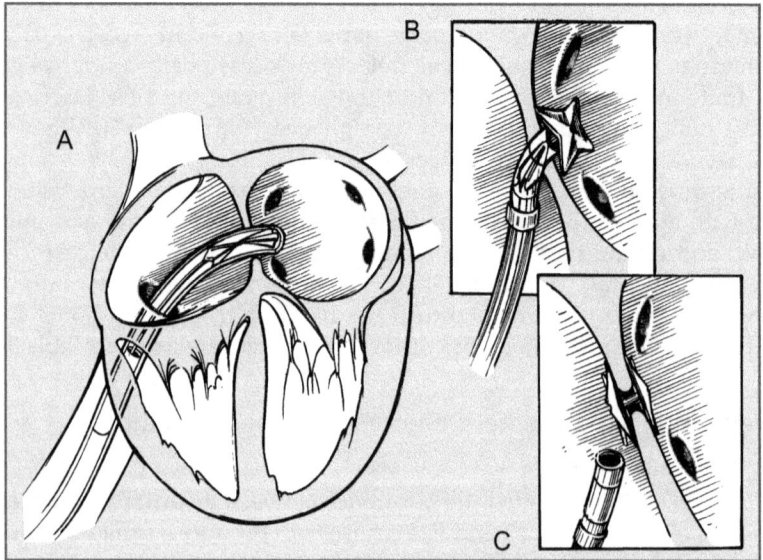

Figure 11-30. Clamshell umbrella occlusion of an ostium secundum atrial septal defect. **A,** A long sheath is positioned in the left atrium. **B,** The distal umbrella arms are opened in the left atrium and the umbrella and sheath are pulled back together to the atrial septum. **C,** The proximal set of arms is then delivered on the right side of the atrial septum. The correct position of the device is confirmed by fluoroscopy, angiography, and echocardiography before the device is released. (From Castañeda AR, Jonas RA, Mayer JE Jr, et al: **Cardiac surgery of the neonate and infant,** Philadelphia, 1994, WB Saunders.)

there is an appreciable delay between the radial and femoral pulses, and the pulsating, engorged intercostal arteries may also be palpable. In an older child the engorged arteries may cause notching of the lower borders of the ribs seen on the chest x-ray film (Figure 11-32). Boys are more likely than girls are to have coarctation of the aorta, but coarctation is present in a significant proportion of individuals with Turner syndrome (see Figure 11-26).

Nature of the Murmur of Coarctation of the Aorta

The systolic murmur of coarctation of the aorta is grade II or III and audible over the aortic and pulmonic areas. A characteristic feature is that the murmur is heard as well or better over the back, because it is generated more deeply in the chest than most other heart murmurs. Because the coarctation murmur is augmented by murmurs in the engorged intercostal vessels, it may be continuous.

Patients with coarctation of the aorta commonly also have a bicuspid aortic valve that produces a murmur that peaks early in systole, is loudest in the second right intercostal space, and is preceded by an ejection sound (Figure 11-33). It may be difficult to distinguish this murmur from the murmur

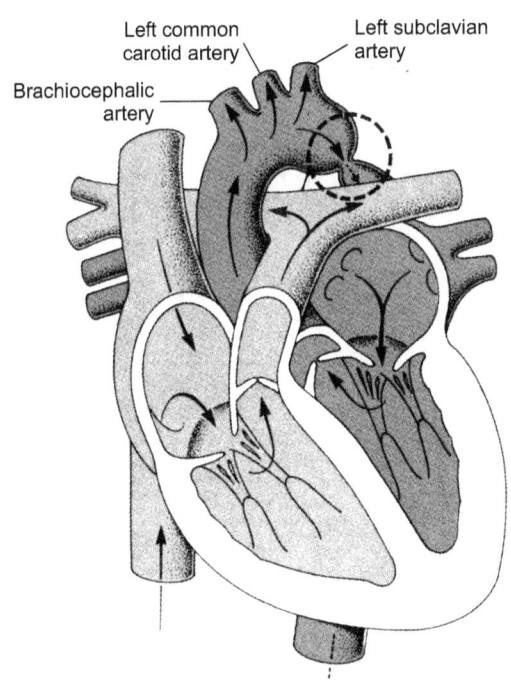

Figure 11-31. Coarctation of the aorta. Flow patterns are normal but are diminished distal to the coarctation. Blood pressure is increased in vessels leaving the aorta proximal to the coarctation. (From Foster R, Hunsberger MM, Anderson JT: **Family-centered nursing care of children,** Philadelphia, 1990, WB Saunders.)

Figure 11-32. Chest x-ray film from a patient with coarctation **(COARC)** of the aorta. Arrows point to sites of notching on the undersurfaces of the posterior ribs. The ascending aorta **(Ao)** forms a rightward convexity. A dilated left subclavian artery **(LSA)** is seen above the coarctation, and a dilated descending aorta **(DA)** is seen below, forming together the silhouette of a "figure 3." (From Perloff JK: **The clinical recognition of congenital heart disease,** ed 4, Philadelphia, 1994, WB Saunders.)

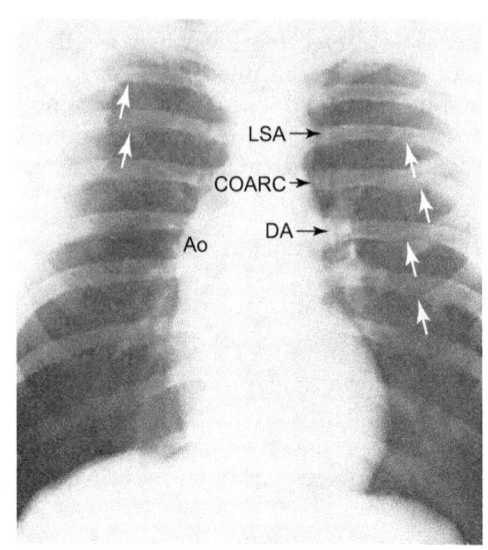

Figure 11-33. Phonocardiograms from a 10-year-old boy with coarctation of the aorta and bicuspid aortic valve. Auscultatory signs of the bicuspid aortic valve are in the tracing from the second right intercostal space **(2RICS),** namely, an aortic ejection sound **(E),** a short midsystolic murmur **(SM),** and an early diastolic murmur **(EDM)** of aortic regurgitation. The tracing from the patient's back was recorded over the site of coarctation and shows a murmur that is delayed in onset and extends well into diastole **(arrows).** (From Perloff JK: **The clinical recognition of congenital heart disease,** ed 4, Philadelphia, 1994, WB Saunders.)

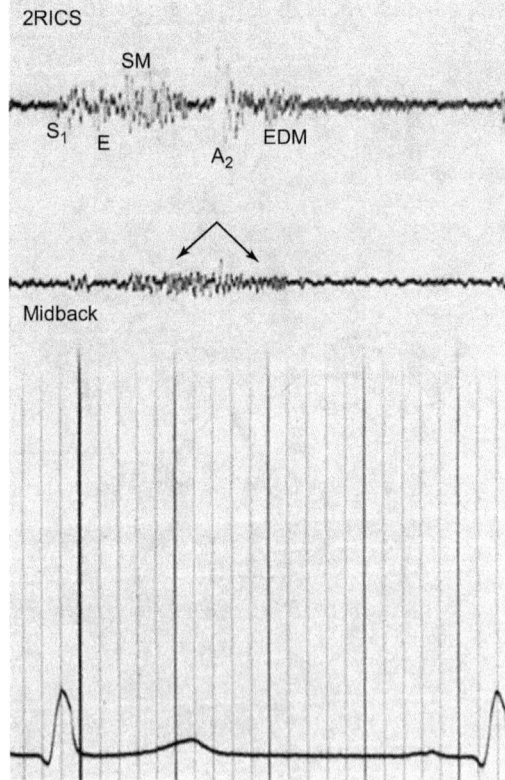

generated by the coarctation itself or, more rarely, by the collateral circulation.

In infancy, coarctation of the aorta is commonly associated with a ventricular septal defect and is discovered because the large shunt, augmented by the coarctation, causes congestive failure. A patent ductus arteriosus is also often present.

COARCTATION OF THE ABDOMINAL AORTA

Coarctation of the abdominal aorta is associated with a systolic murmur audible over the abdomen and lower back. The collateral arteries in the lower intercostal spaces are palpable, and x-ray examination of the chest demonstrates notching of the lower but not the upper ribs. Coarctation of the abdominal aorta is most common in girls and occurs in association with coarctation at the ductus arteriosus (juxtaductal coarctation), the most common site.

BIBLIOGRAPHY

Armstrong WF, Feigenbaum H: Echocardiography. In Braunwald E, Zipes DP, Libby P, editors: **Heart disease,** ed 6, Philadelphia, 2001, WB Saunders.

Braunwald E, Perloff JK: Physical examination of the heart and circulation. In Braunwald E, Zipes DP, Libby P, editors: **Heart disease,** ed 6, Philadelphia, 2001, WB Saunders.

Ehlers KH, Engle MA, Levin AR, et al: Left ventricular abnormality with late mitral insufficiency and abnormal electrocardiogram, **Am J Cardiol** 26(4):333-340, 1970.

Engle MA: Evaluation of systolic murmurs in school-age children, **J Cardiovasc Med** 6(3):217-227, 1981.

Engle MA: Heart sounds and murmurs in diagnosis of heart disease, **Pediatr Ann** 10(3):18-31, 1981.

Engle MA, Ehlers KH: Auscultation and phonocardiography in the recognition and differential diagnosis of congenital aortic stenosis. In Segal B, editor: **Theory and practice of auscultation. Ninth Hahnemann Symposium,** Philadelphia, 1963, FA Davis.

Fiddler GI, Scott O: Heart murmurs audible across the room in children with mitral valve prolapse, **Br Heart J** 44:201-203, 1980.

Friedman WF, Silverman N: Congenital heart disease in infancy and childhood. In Braunwald E, Zipes DP, Libby P, editors: **Heart disease,** ed 6, Philadelphia, 2001, WB Saunders.

Kawabori I, Stevenson JG, Dooley TK, et al: The significance of carotid bruits in children: transmitted murmur of vascular origin, studied by pulsed Doppler ultrasound, **Am Heart J** 98(2):160-167, 1979.

Lee TH: Guidelines: use of echocardiography. In Braunwald E, Zipes DP, Libby P, editors: **Heart disease,** ed 6, Philadelphia, 2001, WB Saunders.

Lembo NJ, Dell'Italia LJ, Crawford MH, et al: Bedside diagnosis of systolic murmurs, **N Engl J Med** 318:1572-1578, 1988.

Levine SA, Harvey WP: **Clinical auscultation of the heart,** ed 2, Philadelphia, 1959, WB Saunders.

Liebman J: Diagnosis and management of heart murmurs in children, **Pediatr Rev**

3(10):321-329, 1982.

Lucas RV: Mitral valve prolapse. In Moller JH, Hoffman JIE, editors: **Pediatric cardiovascular medicine,** Philadelphia, 2000, Churchill Livingston.

McNamara DG: Idiopathic benign mitral leaflet prolapse. The pediatrician's view, **Am J Dis Child** 136:152-156, 1982.

Nadas A, Fyler D: **Pediatric cardiology,** ed 3, Philadelphia, 1972, WB Saunders.

Neutze JM, Calder AL, Gentles TL, et al: Aortic stenosis. In Moller JH, Hoffman JIE, editors: **Pediatric cardiovascular medicine,** Philadelphia, 2000, Churchill Livingston.

Pape KE, Pickering D: Asymmetric crying facies: an index of other congenital abnormalities, **J Pediatr** 81:1, 1972.

Park MK: **Pediatric cardiology for practitioners,** ed 3, St. Louis, 1996, Mosby.

Perloff JK: **The clinical recognition of congenital heart disease,** ed 4, Philadelphia, 1994, WB Saunders.

Ravin A, Craddock LD, Wolf PS, et al: **Auscultation of the heart,** ed 3, Chicago, 1977, Year Book.

Rosenthal A: How to distinguish between innocent and pathologic murmurs in childhood, **Pediatr Clin North Am** 31(6):1229-1240, 1984.

Salzberg AM: Congenital malformation of the lower respiratory tract. In Kendig E, Chernick V, editors: **Disorders of the respiratory tract in children,** ed 4, Philadelphia, 1983, WB Saunders.

Selzer A: Changing aspects of the natural history of valvular aortic stenosis, **N Engl J Med** 317(2):91-98, 1987.

Spray TL: Technique of pulmonary autograft aortic valve replacement in children (the Ross procedure), **Semin Thoracic Cardiovasc Surg** 1:165-177. 1998.

Tilkian A, Conover MB: **Understanding heart sounds and murmurs,** ed 3, Philadelphia, 2001, WB Saunders.

Van Mierop LH: Diseases—congenital anomalies. In Yonkman F, editor: **Heart,** Summit, NJ, 1969, Ciba-Geigy.

Chapter 12

Diastolic Murmurs

Diastolic murmurs are usually pathologic. Although there have been descriptions of innocent diastolic murmurs in children, such murmurs are extremely rare. Diastolic murmurs have been described in children with straight back syndrome (see Chapter 11), probably the result of very mild pulmonary regurgitation. Whenever a diastolic murmur is detected in a child, a careful search for a cardiac pathologic condition should be performed.

Diastolic murmurs are generated across either the atrioventricular valves (in mitral or tricuspid stenosis, which are rarely encountered in pediatric patients) or the semilunar valves (in aortic or pulmonary insufficiency). Diastolic murmurs may also occur as part of a continuous murmur, when there is flow through a vessel during diastole. Examples include patients with patent ductus arteriosus, surgically created aortopulmonary shunts, aortopulmonary window, aortopulmonary collaterals, coarctation of the aorta, peripheral pulmonic stenosis, and coronary artery or sinus of Valsalva fistulas.

AORTIC REGURGITATION

The most common and clinically most important form of aortic valve regurgitation in children is congenital aortic regurgitation caused by a bicuspid valve. Other causes of aortic regurgitation in children include rheumatic heart disease, Marfan syndrome, congenital absence of leaflets, unicuspid valve, quadricuspid valve, or aortic insufficiency from prolapse (bulging of the valve leaflets), which is sometimes associated with a high ventricular septal defect.

Nature of the Murmur of Aortic Regurgitation

The diastolic murmur of aortic regurgitation is high-pitched, blowing, and decrescendo even when loud. In children, the murmur usually becomes louder and longer, with increasing severity of the regurgitation. If a valve cusp is retroverted, the murmur has a musical quality (Figure 12-1). The

161

FIGURE 12-1. Musical diastolic murmur in a patient with aortic regurgitation and retroverted aortic cusp. The musical quality is indicated by the multiple harmonics, which appear as distinct semihorizontal lines. **c.p.s.,** Cycles per second; **DM,** diastolic murmur. (From McKusick VA: **Cardiovascular sound in health and disease,** Baltimore, 1958, Williams & Wilkins.)

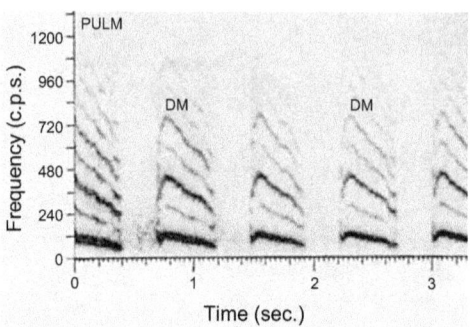

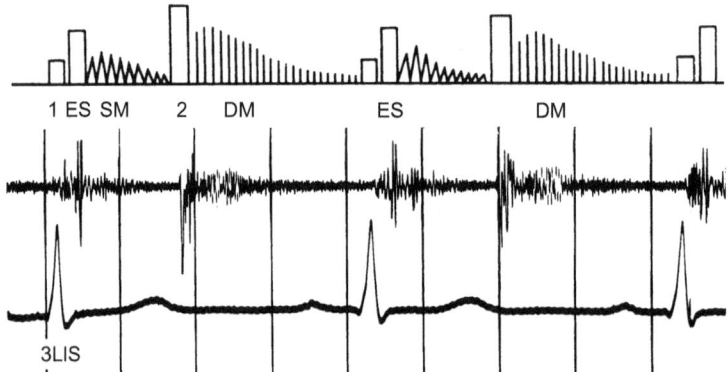

FIGURE 12-2. Diastolic murmur of aortic regurgitation over third left intercostal space **(3LIS).** The high-pitched diastolic murmur **(DM)** starts with the second sound. It is loudest early in diastole and in this case is heard throughout diastole in diminishing intensity. In the diagrammatic representation of this murmur, the diastolic murmur is shown louder than on the phonocardiogram. This is because it is a high-pitched murmur, and high-pitched murmurs seem louder to the ear than when recorded on the phonocardiogram. A moderately loud, medium-pitched systolic murmur **(SM)** is present in this patient. An ejection sound **(ES)** is also present. The second sound is normal or slightly accentuated. (From Ravin A, Craddock L, Wolf PS, et al: **Auscultation of the heart,** ed 3, Chicago, 1977, Year Book.)

murmur begins with the second heart sound and is loudest in early diastole, after which it becomes considerably fainter (Figure 12-2).

The murmur of aortic regurgitation may be missed, because the murmur is often very soft and the patient may not be in the optimal position. Moreover, the murmur can be mistaken for breath sounds because of its high pitch. Auscultation in two positions (with the patient sitting up and leaning forward and with the patient leaning backward, propped on the elbows) may be necessary to hear the murmur of aortic regurgitation. The patient's breath should be held in end expiration. Because the murmur is high-pitched, the diaphragm of the stethoscope should be used. The diaphragm should be pressed firmly against the chest at the third intercostal space over the right and left borders of the sternum, where the murmur is loudest.

In patients with dilatation of the aortic root, deformity of the valve cusps, or dissecting aneurysm of the ascending aorta, the murmur radiates to the right side of the sternum. Palpation of the precordium in patients with severe chronic aortic regurgitation demonstrates a laterally displaced, abnormally forceful left ventricular impulse, which produces a rocking motion of the chest. In severe acute cases, this sign may not be present. It should be possible to feel a systolic thrill over the aortic area as well as over the carotid and subclavian arteries. The thrill is generated by the high velocity of the left ventricular ejection and is associated with a loud systolic murmur.

Additional Clinical Features of Aortic Regurgitation

Although there may not be very much regurgitation through the valve at birth, the degree of regurgitation increases, sometimes slowly and sometimes very suddenly, as the child grows. In addition, the bicuspid valve is very susceptible to bacterial infection (bacterial endocarditis), which may cause rapid destruction of the leaflets and catastrophic failure of the valve. Aortic dissection, a longitudinal cleavage of the medial layer of the vessel, is another complication in 6% of cases in which bicuspid aortic valve is present.

The majority of children with congenital aortic regurgitation are boys. The condition is frequently missed in infancy because of the softness and high pitch of the murmur. If the valve deteriorates gradually, the child may have no symptoms for many years. Some children become aware of neck pulsations or ventricular contractions, especially premature ventricular beats. Other symptoms are vascular pain over the carotid and subclavian arteries, pain over the thoracic or abdominal aorta, and inappropriate sweating.

Patients with aortic regurgitation have an abnormally brisk rise in the arterial pulse, producing the well-known physical sign, the **water hammer** or **Corrigan's pulse.** The water hammer, a toy beloved by children in Victorian England, was made from a sealed glass tube containing water in a vacuum. When the tube was inverted, the water column fell, giving the fingertip against the bottom end a sudden jolt (Figure 12-3).

The pulse of aortic regurgitation is also described as **bounding** or **collapsing.** The pulse pressure is wide, and the diastolic blood pressure is a good index of the severity of aortic insufficiency. In some cases, the pulse may be double peaked (bisferiens). The flushing and blanching caused by the forceful pulsations are even visible in the capillary bed of the fingertips **(Quincke's pulse).**

Differentiating Aortic Regurgitation From Other Conditions

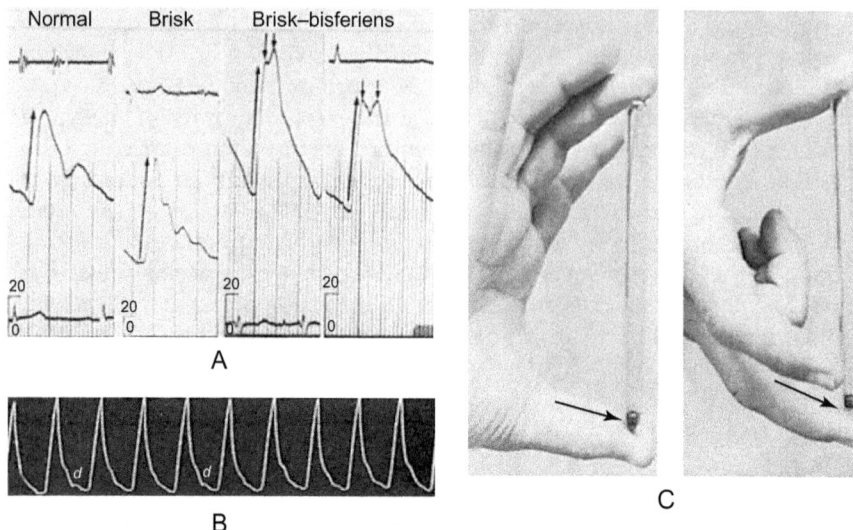

FIGURE 12-3. **A,** Normal brachial arterial pulse for comparison with brachial pulses in moderate to severe pure aortic regurgitation. The latter show a brisk single-peaked pulse and two brisk bisferiens pulses, one with unequal crests and the other with equal crests. **B,** "Pulse of extreme aortic regurgitation" (Mackenzie). **C,** Toy water hammer consisting of a sealed glass tube containing mercury **(arrow)** in a vacuum. As the tube is quickly inverted, the mercury falls abruptly from one end to the other, imparting a jolt or impact to the thumb or fingertip. (From Perloff JK: **Physical examination of the heart and circulation,** ed 3, Philadelphia, 2000, WB Saunders.)

Austin Flint Murmur

In 1862 Dr. Austin Flint described a diastolic murmur at the apex in patients with aortic regurgitation. The murmur is caused by the increased flow of blood across the mitral valve, which occurs because of the increased left ventricular volume needed to allow for normal cardiac output despite significant aortic regurgitation. The murmur begins while the valve is closing and ends at S_1. An Austin Flint murmur is generally indistinguishable from the murmur of mitral stenosis, despite the fact that there is no organic disease of the mitral valve. Thus, the correct diagnosis is usually reached using historical information. It is unlikely for a child in the United States today to have mitral stenosis rather than mitral regurgitation from rheumatic fever.

Occasionally amyl nitrite (an organic drug that causes dilatation of the peripheral vessels) is used to distinguish an Austin Flint murmur from the murmur of mitral stenosis. After a patient inhales amyl nitrite, which decreases the amount of aortic insufficiency, an Austin Flint murmur becomes softer or disappears, but a murmur of mitral stenosis is unaffected.

Relative Aortic Stenosis

Another murmur often heard in cases of aortic insufficiency is a grade II or

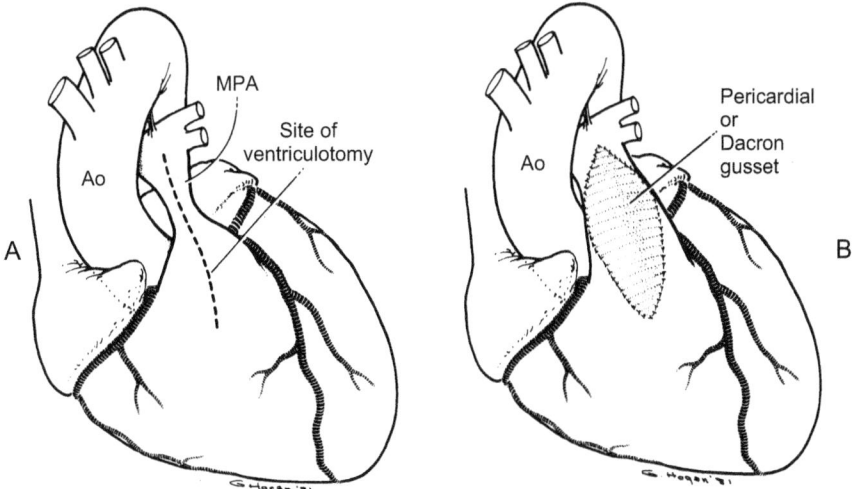

FIGURE 12-4. An incision (ventriculotomy) and a pericardial or Dacron gusset (patch) can be used to enlarge the right ventricular outflow tract during repair of the tetralogy of Fallot or a severe pulmonic stenosis with an intact ventricular septum; this is called a transannular patch. Such a patch always results in some degree of pulmonary regurgitation. **Ao,** Aorta; **MPA,** main pulmonary artery. (From Nugent EW, Plauth WH, Edwards JE, et al: Congenital heart disease. In Hurst JW, editor: **The heart,** ed 6, New York, 1986, McGraw-Hill.)

III ejection murmur of relative aortic stenosis. The murmur results from the increased volume of left ventricular ejection required to ensure a normal cardiac output despite significant aortic regurgitation.

Rheumatic Aortic Insufficiency

Congenital aortic insufficiency is almost always associated with an aortic ejection click. The click allows the examiner to differentiate congenital insufficiency from isolated rheumatic aortic regurgitation, because the latter does not produce a click. The patient's history is also often helpful.

PULMONARY INSUFFICIENCY

There are four causes of pulmonary insufficiency and regurgitation in children. Most commonly, pulmonary insufficiency results from surgery for tetralogy of Fallot, during which a patch is placed across the pulmonary valve annulus to relieve pulmonary stenosis (Figure 12-4). Other causes include congenital abnormality of the pulmonary valve, pulmonary hypertension, and infectious endocarditis.

Nature of the Murmur of Pulmonary Insufficiency

Pulmonary Insufficiency With Hypertension

The murmur of pulmonary insufficiency caused by pulmonary hypertension has the same timing, pitch, and quality as the murmur of aortic regurgitation (see Figure 12-2). It is loudest over the second or third left intercostal space and is best heard with the diaphragm of the stethoscope placed over this area. When loud, the murmur may radiate down the left border of the sternum. It begins just after the second heart sound (Figure 12-5), and the pulmonic component is usually accentuated. Sometimes a pulmonic ejection sound is also present (see Chapter 9).

Congenital or Organic Pulmonary Insufficiency

The murmur of congenital or organic pulmonary insufficiency is a distinctive diastolic murmur. It is low-pitched, crescendo-decrescendo, early in onset, and of short duration (see Figure 12-5). The murmur ends well before the first heart sound and is best heard over the second or third left intercostal space with the bell of the stethoscope.

In patients with a congenital abnormality of the pulmonary valve, one, two, or three cusps may be malformed or even absent. The condition is commonly associated with tetralogy of Fallot. Although the murmur can be detected at birth, usually it is not found until years later. Except in cases of absent pulmonary valve, in which massive dilatation of the pulmonary arteries may produce dramatic early symptoms (associated, for example, with tetralogy of Fallot), pulmonary insufficiency is always associated with pulmonic stenosis.

In mild cases of congenital pulmonary insufficiency, there is little abnormality to see or palpate. In severe cases, there is often a right ventricular

EARLY DIASTOLIC MURMUR

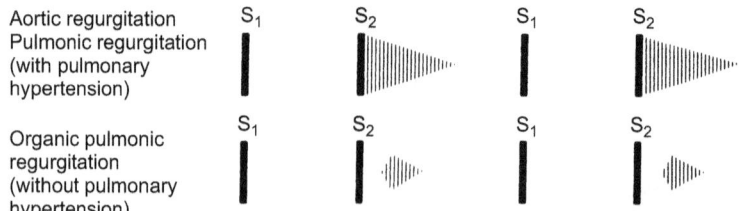

FIGURE 12-5. In aortic regurgitation or pulmonic regurgitation secondary to pulmonary hypertension, the murmur begins almost simultaneously with the second heart sound (S_2). Because the gradient between aorta and left ventricle is maximal almost instantaneously and then slowly decreases, the murmur is also high-pitched and slowly decrescendo. In contrast, organic pulmonary regurgitation without pulmonary hypertension is manifested by a murmur that starts later and has a rapid crescendo with a relatively longer decrescendo. This murmur is lower pitched than the usual early diastolic blowing murmur because regurgitant flow is across a lower pressure system with a small gradient. S_1, First heart sound. (From American Heart Association: **Examination of the heart, Part 4—Auscultation of the heart,** Dallas, 1990, American Heart Association.)

impulse and, occasionally, an impulse over the pulmonary trunk at the second left intercostal space. In addition, the diastolic murmur may produce a palpable thrill over the pulmonary trunk.

Differentiating the Murmurs of Congenital and Hypertensive Pulmonary Insufficiency From Other Murmurs

Hypertensive Versus Congenital or Organic Pulmonary Insufficiency

Figure 12-5 demonstrates the differences between the murmur of pulmonary insufficiency with pulmonary hypertension (or aortic insufficiency) and the murmur of organic pulmonary insufficiency without pulmonary hypertension. The murmur of pulmonary insufficiency with pulmonary hypertension is a long decrescendo murmur beginning just after S_2. In contrast, the murmur of organic pulmonary insufficiency begins well after S_2, is short, crescendo-decrescendo, and ends well before S_1.

Aortic Insufficiency

A diastolic murmur is probably due to aortic insufficiency if the systolic murmur of aortic stenosis is also present (see Chapter 11). Wide transmission of the diastolic murmur also suggests aortic insufficiency, as do bounding pulses and a wide pulse pressure. A diastolic murmur is probably caused by pulmonary insufficiency if it is loud, but the pulse is normal rather than collapsing or bounding. In addition, a loud pulmonic second sound suggests pulmonary insufficiency.

Transannular Patch

As part of the repair of tetralogy of Fallot, a transannular patch (see Figure 12-4) is often used to augment the right ventricular outflow tract. Patients with such patches have a characteristic low-pitched, rumbling, early diastolic murmur of pulmonary insufficiency. This murmur, which is indicative of low pressure in the pulmonary artery, also occurs in cases of congenital absence of the pulmonic valve. It is quite different from the murmur of pulmonary insufficiency with pulmonary hypertension or the murmur of aortic insufficiency (see Figure 12-5).

OTHER DIASTOLIC MURMURS
Active Rheumatic Carditis

Although a systolic murmur is the most frequent finding in children with acute rheumatic fever and carditis, a middiastolic rumbling murmur may also be heard. The murmur **(Carey-Coombs murmur)** is generated by stiffening of the mitral valve cusps, rather than by organic mitral stenosis, which takes years to develop. The Carey-Coombs murmur also has a presystolic component. Both the middiastolic and presystolic murmurs disappear as the inflammation subsides and the heart size diminishes.

Inactive Rheumatic Heart Disease With Significant Mitral Regurgitation

Children with significant mitral regurgitation and a large left ventricle can have a middiastolic murmur even without the presence of mitral stenosis (Figure 12-6). The murmur is generated by increased flow through the mitral valve and enlargement of the left ventricle. The following points distinguish the middiastolic murmur of inactive rheumatic heart disease with significant mitral regurgitation from the middiastolic murmur of mitral stenosis:

1. A child with significant mitral regurgitation generally has little mitral stenosis. Therefore, a diastolic murmur in this child is probably caused by inactive rheumatic heart disease with significant mitral regurgitation.
2. The first heart sound is not accentuated in children with the murmur of inactive rheumatic heart disease with significant mitral regurgitation. In contrast, the first heart sound is accentuated in children with mitral stenosis.
3. An opening snap of the mitral valve (see Chapter 9) is rarely heard in children with the murmur of inactive rheumatic heart disease

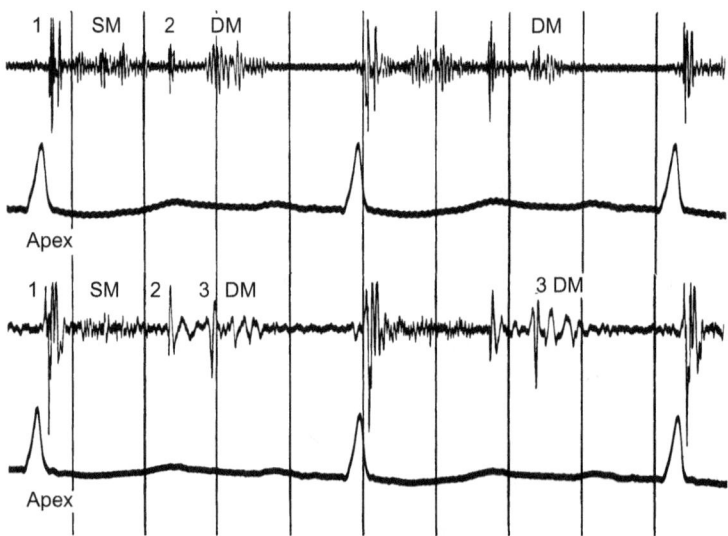

FIGURE 12-6. Middiastolic murmur in a patient with mitral regurgitation. **Upper tracing,** The first sound is followed by a systolic murmur **(SM).** The second sound is of normal intensity. A moderately loud middiastolic murmur **(DM)** is present. **Lower tracing,** In a slightly different area at the apex and with a different method of recording, it is evident that there is a loud third sound (3) followed by a diastolic rumble **(DM).** (From Ravin A, Craddock LD, Wolf P, et al: **Auscultation of the heart,** ed 3, Chicago, 1977, Year Book.)

with significant mitral regurgitation. An opening snap is heard in children with mitral stenosis.

MITRAL STENOSIS

Causes of Mitral Stenosis

Mitral stenosis is not common in children or adolescents. Mitral stenosis is usually caused by rheumatic heart disease resulting from rheumatic fever, and it may take years for sufficient damage to produce symptoms. Once a common cause of mitral stenosis, rheumatic fever is now uncommon in the United States, although its incidence is on the rise.

Rarely, infants and young children have congenital mitral stenosis (not the small mitral orifice that is part of the hypoplastic left heart syndrome), which may be accompanied by coarctation of the aorta and valvular stenosis. Three other common congenital abnormalities (ventricular septal defect, patent ductus arteriosus, and mitral insufficiency) may cause increased flow across a normal mitral valve, generating a middiastolic rumbling murmur. In moderately severe cases of mitral insufficiency, a rumble of relative mitral stenosis may be audible if the annulus is not very dilated. A mitral diastolic murmur may also be heard in conjunction with aortic insufficiency.

Origin of the Murmur of Mitral Stenosis

The murmur of mitral stenosis is caused by the flow of blood through the narrowed mitral orifice during diastole. Because the flow velocity of the blood is relatively low, the murmur is low-pitched and is perceived as a rumble. As the degree of stenosis increases, the filling of the ventricle becomes slower, and the murmur lengthens, permitting an estimation of the degree of stenosis. A patient with mild stenosis has a short middiastolic murmur, whereas a patient with more severe stenosis has a longer murmur (Figure 12-7).

Nature of the Murmur of Mitral Stenosis

The murmur of mitral stenosis is a low-frequency, middiastolic rumble. It is associated with an opening snap and a loud S_1 (Figure 12-8). The opening snap is a short, sharp, high-pitched sound audible in early diastole, 0.04 to 0.12 second after A_2 (see Chapter 9). The loud S_1 is discussed in detail in Chapter 6.

Toward the end of diastole, as the mitral leaflets close, the mitral orifice narrows further. This narrowing causes increased blood flow velocity and produces a presystolic crescendo murmur, ending with the first heart sound (see Figure 12-8). In the past, atrial contraction was thought to cause the presystolic murmur. The theory that the presystolic murmur is caused by mitral closure is supported by the fact that the murmur is audible in patients

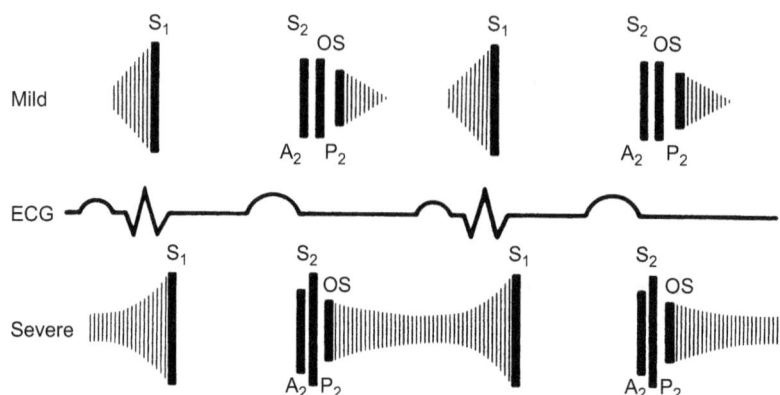

DIASTOLIC FILLING MURMUR (RUMBLE)
Mitral Stenosis

FIGURE 12-7. In mild mitral stenosis, the diastolic gradient across the valve is limited to two phases of rapid ventricular filling in early diastole and presystole. A rumble occurs during either or both periods. As the stenotic process becomes severe, a large gradient exists across the valve during the entire diastolic filling period, and a rumble persists throughout diastole. As the left atrial pressure becomes higher, the time from aortic valve closure sound **(A₂)** to opening snap **(OS)** shortens. In severe mitral stenosis, secondary pulmonary hypertension results in a louder pulmonic valve closure sound **(P₂)** and the splitting interval usually narrows. S_1, First heart sound; S_2, second heart sound. (From American Heart Association: **Examination of the heart, Part 4, Auscultation of the heart,** Dallas, 1990, American Heart Association.)

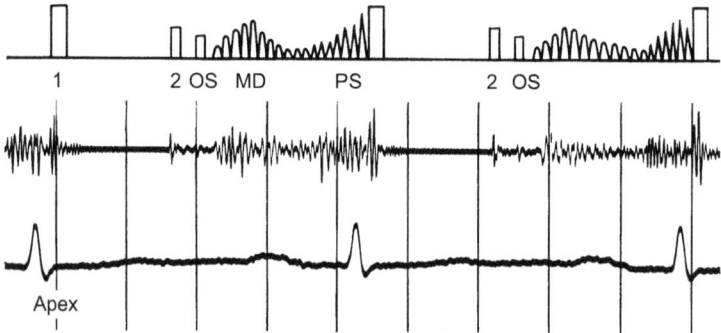

FIGURE 12-8. Diastolic murmur of mitral stenosis. The second sound is followed by a faint opening snap **(OS)**. Diastole is long, and the middiastolic murmur **(MD)** begins to fade before the presystolic murmur **(PS)**. The presystolic murmur has been attributed to atrial contraction, although recent studies identified the murmur in patients with atrial fibrillation and no atrial contraction. (From Ravin A, Craddock D, Wolf PS, et al: **Auscultation of the heart,** ed 3, Chicago, 1977, Year Book.)

who are in atrial fibrillation and who do not have atrial contraction.

The murmur of mitral stenosis is heard most easily with the patient lying on the left side. Because the murmur is low-pitched, the bell of the stethoscope should be used. The murmur is audible in only a very circumscribed area, just over the point of maximum impulse. Therefore, after carefully palpating for this point, the examiner should place the bell over it lightly. If the bell is moved only slightly from the point of maximum impulse, the murmur may not be heard.

TRICUSPID STENOSIS
Nature of the Murmur of Tricuspid Stenosis

Tricuspid stenosis produces a rumbling diastolic murmur that is very difficult to differentiate from the murmur of mitral stenosis, except by its location. It is easiest to hear the murmur of tricuspid stenosis with the

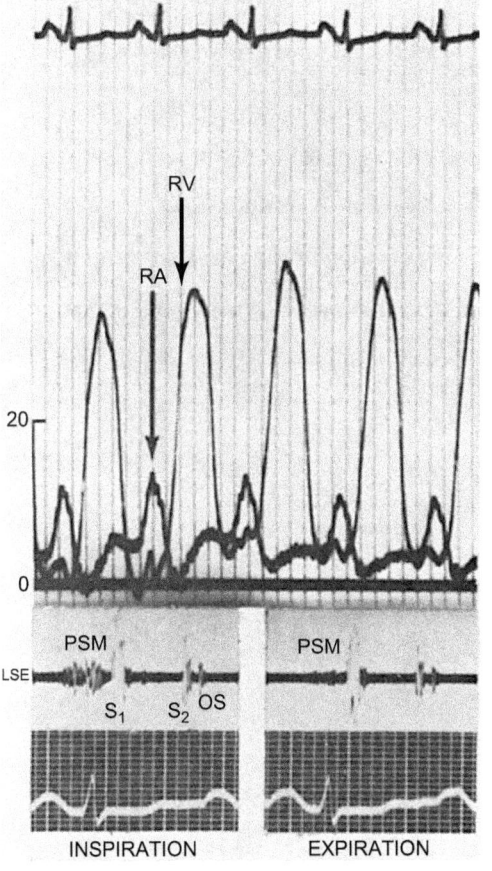

FIGURE 12-9. The presystolic murmur of tricuspid stenosis. **Upper tracing,** Right atrial **(RA)** and right ventricular **(RV)** pressure pulse tracings in a patient with rheumatic tricuspid stenosis. During inspiration the gradient increases as right ventricular diastolic pressure falls and right atrial pressure rises. **Lower tracing,** The presystolic murmur of tricuspid stenosis is accentuated by inspiration and decreases during expiration in parallel with the gradient. **LSE,** Left sternal edge; **OS,** opening snap; **PSM,** presystolic murmur. (From Perloff JK: The physiologic mechanisms of cardiac and vascular signs, **J Am Coll Cardiol** 1:196, 1983.)

patient recumbent, using the bell of the stethoscope, placed just to the left of the lower end of the sternum (tricuspid area). Sometimes the murmur is also heard well at the lower right sternal border. It is important that only very gentle pressure be applied to the bell.

Differentiating the Murmur of Tricuspid Stenosis From the Murmur of Mitral Stenosis

Like the murmur of tricuspid regurgitation (see Chapter 11), the murmur of tricuspid stenosis becomes louder on inspiration. This respiratory variation allows differentiation from the murmur of mitral stenosis, which is unaffected by respiration. In addition, the murmur of tricuspid stenosis is often higher pitched and scratchier than the murmur of mitral stenosis (Figure 12-9). The murmur of relative tricuspid stenosis is important in the diagnosis of large atrial septal defect.

BIBLIOGRAPHY

Criley JM, Hermer AJ: The crescendo presystolic murmur of mitral stenosis with atrial fibrillation, **N Engl J Med** 285:1284, 1971.

Papadopoulos GS, Folger GM: Diastolic murmurs in the newborn of a benign nature, **Int J Cardiol** 3:107-109, 1983.

Perloff JK: **The clinical recognition of congenital heart disease,** ed 4, Philadelphia, 1994, WB Saunders.

Perloff JK: **Physical examination of the heart and circulation,** ed 3, Philadelphia, 2000, WB Saunders.

Ravin A, Craddock LD, Wolf PS, et al: **Auscultation of the heart,** ed 3, Chicago, 1977, Year Book.

Tilkian A, Conover M: **Understanding heart sounds,** ed 3, Philadelphia, 2001, WB Saunders.

Chapter 13

Continuous Murmurs

Most continuous murmurs are not audible throughout the cardiac cycle. Rather, they begin in systole and extend into diastole. A midsystolic to late systolic augmentation of a continuous murmur imparts a mechanical quality to the sound, and such murmurs are called **machinery murmurs.**

With the exception of the mammary souffle and the venous hum (see Chapter 11), continuous murmurs are a pathologic finding. A continuous murmur can be produced in three ways:

1. **Rapid blood flow.** The venous hum and mammary souffle result from rapid blood flow.
2. **High-to-low pressure shunting.** When blood is shunted from the arterial to the venous circulation, a continuous murmur is produced. The murmur of patent ductus arteriosus is produced by such shunting.
3. **Localized arterial obstruction.** Some patients with coarctation of the aorta, peripheral pulmonic stenosis, or obstruction of a large artery (e.g., the femoral) have a continuous murmur.

TO-AND-FRO MURMURS

An examiner must be able to distinguish continuous murmurs from to-and-fro murmurs. To-and-fro murmurs (which occur in patients with two simultaneous valvular abnormalities, such as aortic stenosis and aortic insufficiency) are composed of both a systolic and a diastolic murmur, which combine to produce a distinctive sound. A comparison of a continuous murmur and a to-and-fro murmur is presented in Figure 13-1. .

PATENT DUCTUS ARTERIOSUS

In a normal full-term infant, the ductus begins to close just after birth. Closure is complete by the second week of life. By the third week, the ductus should be permanently sealed. A patent ductus arteriosus, most common in

CONTINUOUS MURMUR VS. TO-FRO MURMUR

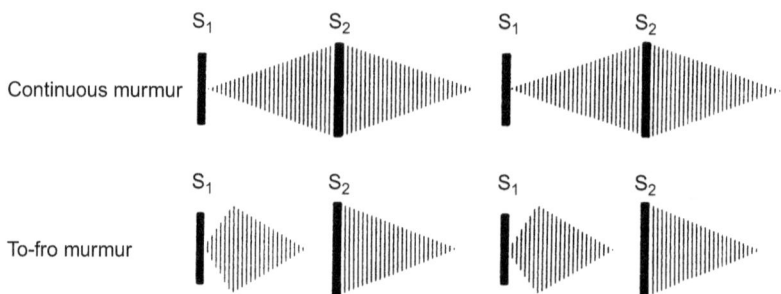

FIGURE 13-1. During abnormal communication between high-pressure and low-pressure systems, a large pressure gradient exists throughout the cardiac cycle, producing a continuous murmur. A classic example is patent ductus arteriosus. At times this type of murmur is confused with a to-and-fro murmur, which is a combination of a systolic ejection murmur and a murmur of semilunar valve incompetence. A classic example of a to-and-fro murmur is aortic stenosis and regurgitation. A continuous murmur builds to crescendo around the second heart sound **(S_2)**, whereas a to-and-fro murmur has two components. The midsystolic ejection component decrescendos and disappears as it approaches S_2. **S_1,** First heart sound. (From Shaver JA, Leonard JL, deLeon DF: **Examination of the heart. Part 4, Auscultation of the heart,** Dallas, 1990, American Heart Association.)

preterm (premature) infants, is caused by the persistence of the normal fetal vascular channel between the pulmonary artery and the aorta (Figure 13-2) (see Chapter 1).

A second type of abnormal connection, the **aortopulmonary window,** develops when the septum between the aorta and pulmonary artery does not fully form. An aortopulmonary window is almost always very large and rarely may either have the continuous murmur characteristic of patent ductus arteriosus or, like patent ductus arteriosus, a systolic murmur that can be confused with a ventricular septal defect.

Diagnosis of Patent Ductus Arteriosus

A characteristic pattern occurs in the discovery of the presence of a patent ductus arteriosus. Usually, the newborn infant is examined, pronounced normal, and sent home as a healthy baby. As neonatal pulmonary vascular resistance falls, blood begins to flow from the aorta to the pulmonary artery through the ductus, and the typical murmur develops. Thus, the diagnosis is made at the first well-baby examination. One must remember that patency of the ductus is normal in the newborn (first 24 hours of life), but that a few weeks later a patent ductus is abnormal.

Patent ductus arteriosus is more common in girls (sex ratio, 3:2), tends to affect siblings, and may be a complication of maternal rubella. In addition, because the higher oxygen levels at sea level are a potent constrictor of the

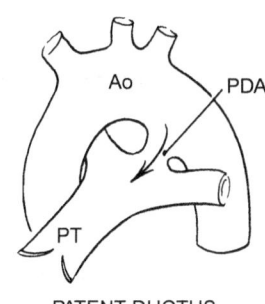

PATENT DUCTUS

FIGURE 13-2. Patent ductus arteriosus **(PDA)** and aortopulmonary window **(APW).** The aortic end of the ductus lies immediately beyond the origin of the left subclavian artery. The pulmonary orifice of the ductus is located immediately to the left of the bifurcation of the pulmonary trunk **(PT).** An aortopulmonary window consists of a round or oval communication between adjacent parts of the ascending aorta **(Ao)** and pulmonary trunk. The ligamentum arteriosum **(Lig. Art.)** is shown as a landmark. (From Perloff JK: **The clinical recognition of congenital heart disease,** ed 4, Philadelphia, 1994, WB Saunders.)

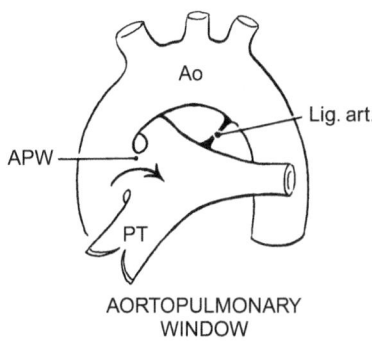

AORTOPULMONARY WINDOW

ductus, patent ductus arteriosus is six times more common in children born at high altitudes. Patent ductus is much more common in premature infants than in full-term infants.

Nature of the Murmur of Patent Ductus Arteriosus

The characteristic murmur of a patent ductus arteriosus is continuous. The murmur is louder during systole and persists, without interruption, through the second heart sound, which it envelops, becoming softer during diastole (Figure 13-3), in contrast with the typical venous hum. The murmur of patent ductus arteriosus has a peculiar machinery-like quality.

In the newborn, because of relatively high pulmonary vascular resistance, one often hears only the systolic component of the murmur, making diagnosis difficult. Thereafter the diastolic component usually becomes audible. There is a crude relationship between the amplitude of the murmur and the size of the ductal opening: in general, the louder the murmur, the larger the ductal opening.

The murmur is best heard over the first and second left intercostal spaces, adjacent to the sternum, where it is loudest (Figure 13-4). Both the bell and the diaphragm of the stethoscope should be used. If the systolic component of the murmur is loud, it may be audible along the left sternal

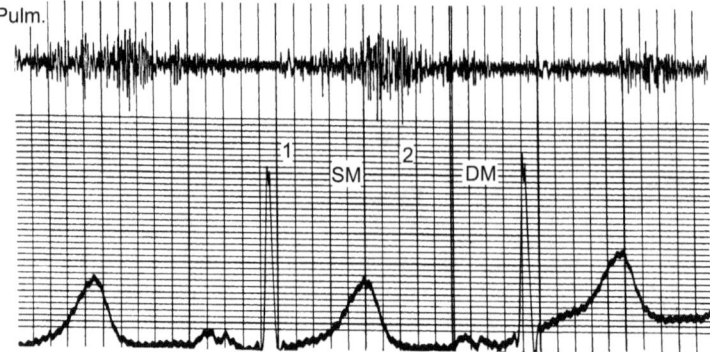

FIGURE 13-3. Continuous murmur of patent ductus arteriosus. Note that the murmur completely envelops S₂ and that there is a late systolic crescendo. **DM,** Diastolic murmur; **SM,** systolic murmur. (From Nadas AS, Fyler DC: **Pediatric cardiology,** ed 3, Philadelphia, 1972, WB Saunders. Copyright AS Nadas.)

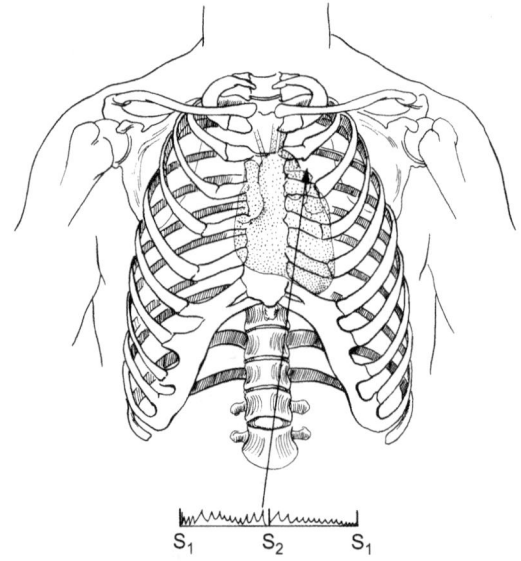

FIGURE 13-4. The murmur of patent ductus arteriosus and where the murmur is best heard.

edge and sometimes the apex. The softer diastolic component is transmitted less well. Occasionally the systolic component can be heard over the back in the interscapular area. In some patients with patent ductus arteriosus, the murmur is loud and harsh at the lower left sternal border, making it difficult to rule out an associated ventricular septal defect.

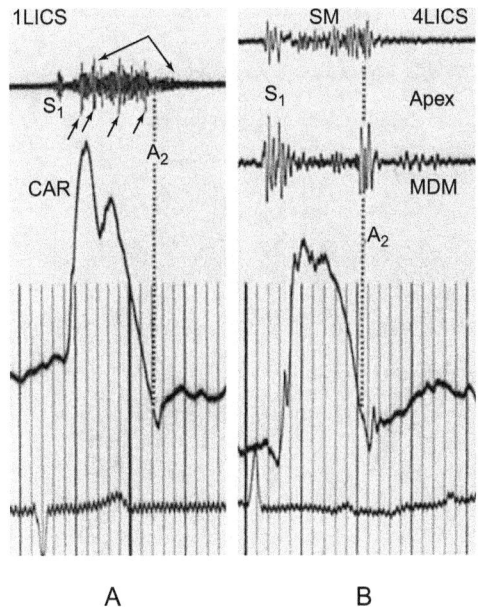

FIGURE 13-5. Tracings from an 18-year-old woman with a large patent ductus arteriosus, pulmonary hypertension, and persistent 2.3-to-1 left-to-right shunt. **A,** In the first left intercostal space **(1LICS),** the ductus murmur is shortened but remains continuous **(upper arrows).** Eddy sounds punctuate the murmur **(lower arrows). B,** At the fourth left intercostal space **(4LICS),** there is a holosystolic murmur that is devoid of eddy sounds. At the apex there is a short, low-frequency middiastolic murmur **(MDM)** caused by augmented mitral valve flow. **CAR,** Carotid pulse, **SM,** systolic murmur. (From Perloff JK: **The clinical recognition of congenital heart disease,** ed 4, Philadelphia, 1994, WB Saunders.)

Pulmonary Vascular Disease and Pulmonary Hypertension

Although unusual, patent ductus may be complicated by pulmonary vascular disease and pulmonary hypertension. If these complications develop at all, they usually do not occur until late childhood. As pulmonary vascular resistance rises, diastolic flow through the ductus diminishes and may even cease. This causes the diastolic component of the murmur to disappear, leaving only a holosystolic murmur (Figure 13-5). If pulmonary vascular resistance increases, left-to-right shunting ceases and no murmur is audible. In severe cases, right-to-left shunting, with no associated murmur, is present, as in ventricular septal defect with Eisenmenger syndrome.

Additional Physical Findings

Several important findings may be detected during physical examination of a child with patent ductus arteriosus. A brisk, bounding peripheral pulse is an important clue to the diagnosis, especially in an ill newborn without the typical murmur. The arterial pulse rises rapidly to a single peak or twin peaks then quickly collapses (Figure 13-6).

If the ductus is large, there may be vigorous precordial activity in an infant, obvious to the mother when she holds the child against her chest. The examiner is often able to palpate a systolic thrill over the sternal notch and the second and third intercostal spaces just to the left of the sternum. In addition to the bounding pulses, there may be symptoms of congestive heart failure, as in other left-to-right shunts in infancy. A surprisingly good pulse

NORMAL ◄─────── PATENT DUCTUS ───────►

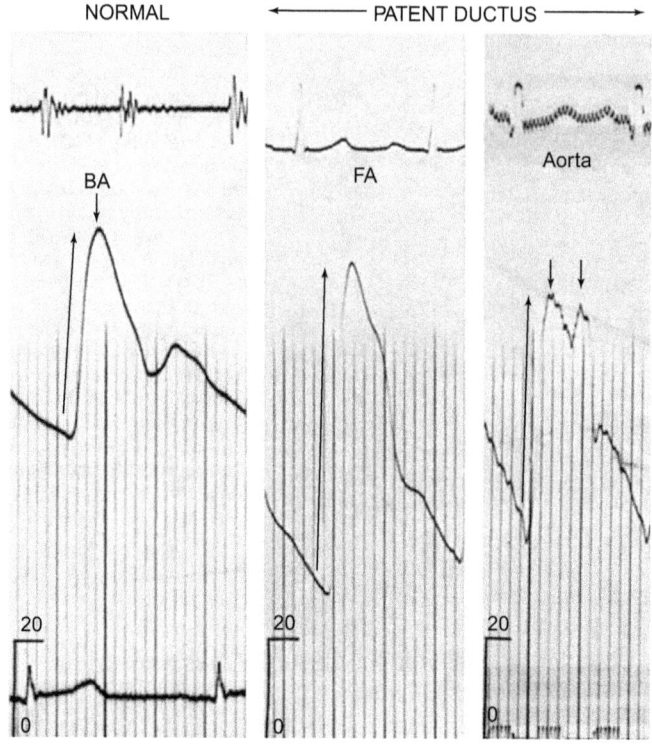

FIGURE 13-6. Pulses from the femoral artery **(FA)** and aorta in two patients, age 18 months and 22 months, with patent ductus arteriosus and large left-to-right shunts. The pulses exhibit a brisk rate of rise, a single or bisferiens (twin) peak, a rapid collapse, and a wide pulse pressure. A normal systemic brachial arterial pulse **(BA)** is shown for comparison. (From Perloff JK: **The clinical recognition of congenital heart disease,** ed 4, Philadelphia, 1994,

in an infant with congestive failure should suggest patent ductus arteriosus.

Harrison's grooves may be present if there is a large amount of blood flowing from the aorta to the pulmonary artery through the ductus. If the child is underdeveloped, the examiner should search for other signs (such as cataracts, deafness, or mental retardation) that might indicate a maternal rubella infection. If trisomy 18 is present, the child may have rocker bottom feet, overlapping fingers, and lax skin as well as additional cardiac abnormalities (Figure 13-7).

If congestive heart failure does not develop within the first year of life, most children with patent ductus arteriosus do not have symptoms unless pulmonary vascular disease and pulmonary hypertension develop.

Pulmonary Vascular Disease and Pulmonary Hypertension

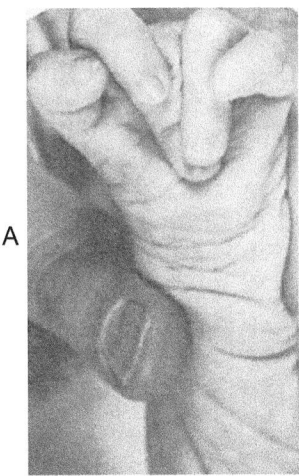
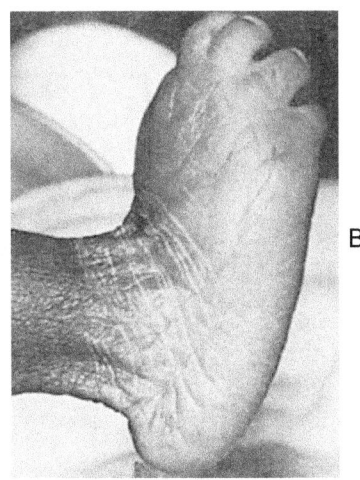

A

B

FIGURE 13-7. A, The hand of an infant girl with trisomy 18 and patent ductus arteriosus with ventricular septal defect. The fingers bend and overlap (clinodactyly), and the skin is lax. **B,** The "rocker bottom" foot of a 6-week-old cyanotic boy with trisomy 16-18 and right ventricle origin of both great arteries with supracristal ventricular septal defect. (From Perloff JK: **Physical examination of the heart and circulation,** ed 3, Philadelphia, 2000, WB Saunders.)

If this relatively rare complication occurs, the patient usually complains of fatigue during exertion. Sometimes the pulmonary trunk enlarges and causes hoarseness because of compression of the recurrent laryngeal nerve. In severe cases, there is shunting of poorly oxygenated blood to the lower extremities (Figure 13-8). The desaturated blood in the pulmonary artery passes through the ductus and enters the aorta at or immediately beyond the left subclavian artery, the last vessel supplying the upper extremities. In one young patient reported by Perloff (1994), this condition **(differential cyanosis)** became evident when she bathed. In a tub of warm water, the girl noticed that her toes were blue but her fingers were pink. There was no murmur, and the loud P_2 invariably present in pulmonary hypertension was overlooked.

Differentiating the Murmur of Patent Ductus Arteriosus From Other Murmurs

The envelopment of the second heart sound is an important characteristic of the murmur of patent ductus arteriosus. If such envelopment does not occur, the murmur in question probably is not that of patent ductus arteriosus. Also, in patients with a large patent ductus, the examiner may hear a diastolic rumble at the cardiac apex, which may be mistaken for the murmur of mitral stenosis and, as in ventricular septal defect, simply reflects increased flow through a normal mitral valve.

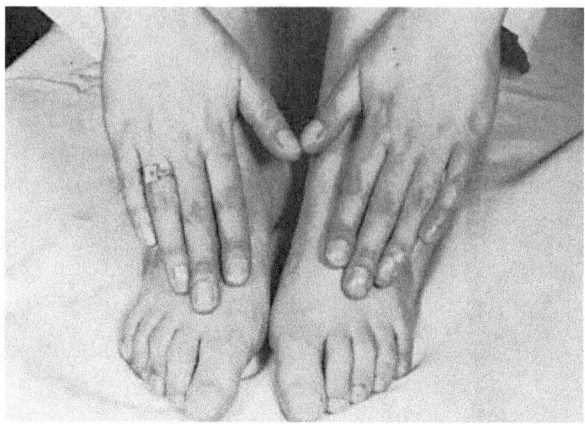

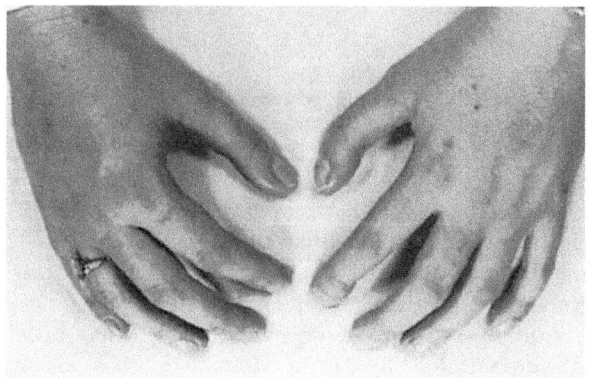

FIGURE 13-8. Differential cyanosis in a case of patent ductus arteriosus with pulmonary hypertension. Photographs of a 28-year-old woman with reversed shunt. In the upper picture, she is sitting in bed with her hands placed on the dorsum of her feet. The right hand is acyanotic, and the fingers are not clubbed. The left hand exhibits mild cyanosis with clubbing (compare the thumbs). The toes are cyanosed and clubbed. The lower picture is a close-up of the hands. Moderate clubbing and cyanosis are present in the left hand but not the right (compare the thumbs). Only the left is clubbed. (From Perloff JK: **The clinical recognition of congenital heart disease,** ed 4, Philadelphia, 1994, WB Saunders.)

Ventricular Septal Defect

In an infant, patent ductus may be difficult to differentiate from ventriular septal defect (see Chapter 11). A bounding arterial pulse suggests patent ductus arteriosus.

Venous Hum

The murmur of venous hum (see Chapter 11) may sound like the murmur of patent ductus arteriosus. Venous hum is loudest above the clavicle and is abolished by compressing the jugular vein. In contrast, the murmur of patent ductus arteriosus is loudest at the second intercostal space to the left of the sternum, and jugular vein compression does not abolish it. In addition, a venous hum is usually louder during diastole.

Tetralogy of Fallot

Tetralogy of Fallot (see Chapter 15) with severe pulmonary stenosis or atresia may generate a continuous murmur, even though the ductus is not patent. In these patients, the continuous murmur results from the flow of blood through dilated, tortuous bronchial arteries. Patients with tetralogy of Fallot have central cyanosis (cyanosis involving the whole body), and those with patent ductus do not. If the bronchial arteries are large, only when pulmonary vascular disease and hypertension develop do patients with patent ductus arteriosus become cyanotic, and the cyanosis usually involves only part of the body. However, the cyanosis may not be visible, especially if the patient is dark skinned.

Prognosis

After successful surgical closure, patent ductus arteriosus may be considered cured.

PERICARDIAL FRICTION RUB
Origin of the Pericardial Friction Rub

A pericardial friction rub occurs when there is inflammation of the pericardial membrane, a relatively common occurrence after surgery and inflammatory diseases, such as rheumatic fever and rheumatoid arthritis. The roughened part of the pericardium in contact with the heart (the visceral pericardium or epicardium) rubs against the outer pericardial layer (the parietal pericardium) and generates the characteristic creaking sound. In patients with pericarditis and a friction rub, the sound has three components. The first is presystolic and is produced by atrial contraction. The second is systolic and associated with ventricular contraction. The third is diastolic and results from rapid ventricular filling (Figure 13-9).

Nature of the Pericardial Friction Rub

A pericardial friction rub, which sounds like the creaking of leather, is best heard with the stethoscope placed over the left sternal border, where the rub is most audible. It is loudest during inspiration, although the intensity is extremely variable, changing from one moment to the next. In addition, the amplitude of the rub varies with position, and the examiner should listen to the patient in several positions—sitting, lying down, and standing.

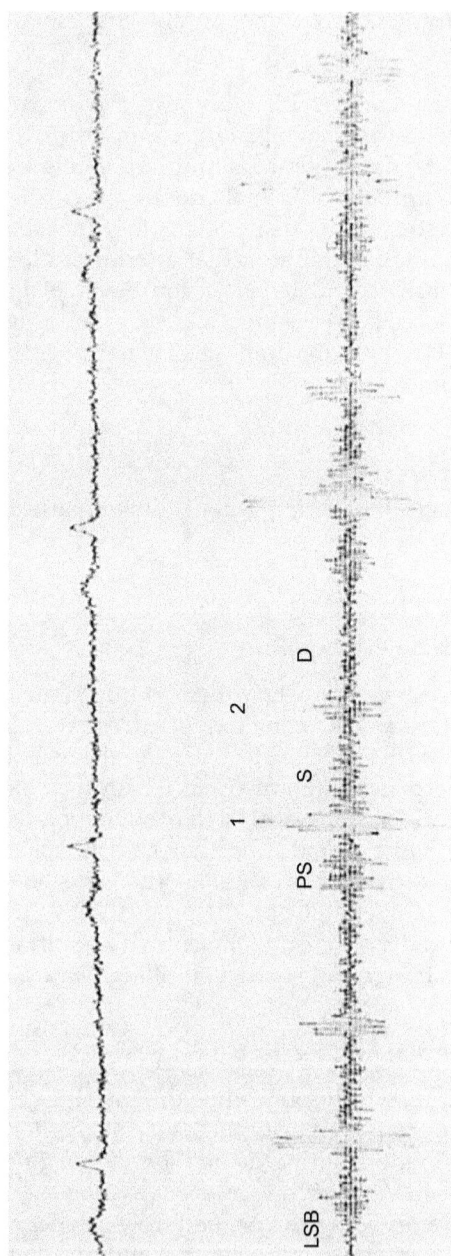

FIGURE 13-9. Pericardial friction rub. **D,** Diastolic; **LSB,** left sternal border; **PS,** presystolic component; **S,** systolic. (From Ravin A, Craddock D, Wolf PS, et al: **Auscultation of the heart,** ed 3, Chicago, 1977, Year Book.)

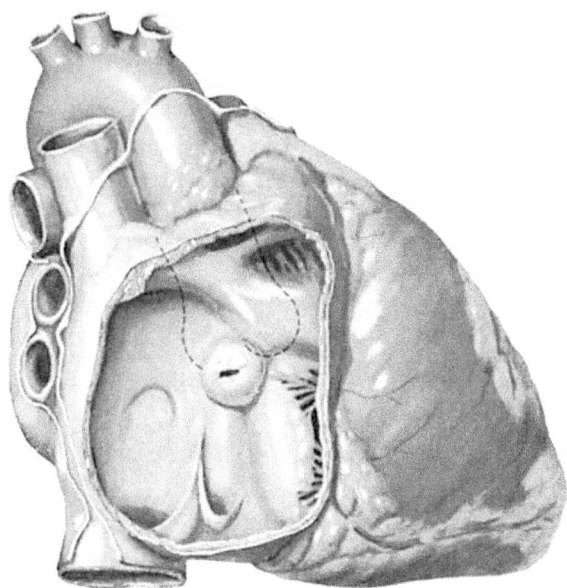

FIGURE 13-10. Sinus of Valsalva aneurysm. (From Van Mierop LHS: Diseases—congenital anomalies. In Yonkman F, editor: **The heart,** Summit, NJ, 1969, Ciba-Geigy.)

Differentiating Pericardial Friction Rub From Other Sounds

Pleural Friction Rub
Like the pericardial friction rub, the pleural friction rub generates sounds with a creaking-leather quality. However, the pleural friction rub has a respiratory rhythm that is audible during inspiration and expiration.

Mediastinal Crunch
The mediastinal crunch (Hamman's sign) is produced by free air in the mediastinum. The sound has a high-pitched crackling quality and often coincides with ventricular systole.

Multiple Systolic Clicks
These sounds, associated with mitral valve prolapse, may sometimes be confused with a pericardial friction rub.

Artifact
Poor auscultatory technique may result in friction of skin or clothing on the diaphragm of the stethoscope, simulating a friction rub.

OTHER CONTINUOUS MURMURS
Arteriovenous Fistula

This type of abnormal connection between an artery and a vein can affect any vessel—bronchial, pleural, pulmonary, coronary, intercostal, abdominal, or cerebral. One example is a sinus of Valsalva aneurysm (Figure 13-10), which can form an abnormal connection to the right side of the heart if the aneurysm should rupture. Generally, the rupture occurs in a young adult, and heart failure develops rapidly. The clinical picture is dramatic, with the patient experiencing shortness of breath, chest pain, bounding pulses, and the new onset of a machinery-like, continuous murmur associated with a thrill over the lower precordial area.

Local Arterial Obstruction

Occasionally the narrowing of a large artery, such as the brachiocephalic or femoral, can generate a continuous murmur.

BIBLIOGRAPHY

Friedman WF, Silverman N: Congenital heart disease in infancy and childhood. In Braunwald E, Zipes DP, Libby P, editors: **Heart disease,** ed 6, Philadelphia, 2001, WB Saunders.

Perloff JK: **The clinical recognition of congenital heart disease,** ed 4, Philadelphia, 1994, WB Saunders.

Ravin A, Craddock LD, Wolf PS, et al: **Auscultation of the heart,** ed 3, Chicago, 1977, Year Book.

Tilkian A, Conover MB: **Understanding heart sounds,** ed 3, Philadelphia, 2001, WB Saunders.

Van Mierop LHS: Diseases—congenital anomalies. In Yonkman F, editor: **The heart,** Summit, NJ, 1969, Ciba-Geigy.

Chapter 14

Surgically Created Shunts and Prosthetic Valves

SHUNTS

Blalock-Taussig Shunt

The Blalock-Taussig operation was the first procedure used for tetralogy of Fallot. It is an end-to-side subclavian artery to pulmonary artery shunt, which is still employed (Figure 14-1). In an alternative procedure used more commonly, the **modified Blalock-Taussig procedure,** a Gore-Tex tube is used to connect the pulmonary artery to the subclavian artery. The advantages of the modified procedure are that it is not necessary to sacrifice the subclavian artery, that the size of the shunt can be controlled precisely, and that there are fewer problems (such as kinking or stenosis) with the distal pulmonary artery. The disadvantages of the modified procedure are those associated with any foreign material; that is, a higher rate of thrombosis and occlusion and a higher risk of endocarditis.

In a very sick infant, a **central aortopulmonary shunt** may be constructed. This is a quick procedure in which a piece of Gore-Tex tubing is used to connect the aorta and the pulmonary artery.

The Murmur of the Blalock-Taussig Shunt

A Blalock-Taussig shunt generates a continuous murmur, audible under the clavicle on the side of the shunt or over the operative scar. If pulmonary vascular resistance is high, or if the shunt is small, the murmur is heard only in systole. The **central shunt** also generates a continuous murmur, usually easily audible over the center of the chest.

A change over time in the murmur of a Blalock-Taussig shunt is a clue to occlusion or narrowing of the shunt. The most common change with shunt narrowing is loss of the diastolic component of the murmur. However, in a large shunt, loss of the diastolic murmur can occur because of an increase in pulmonary vascular resistance.

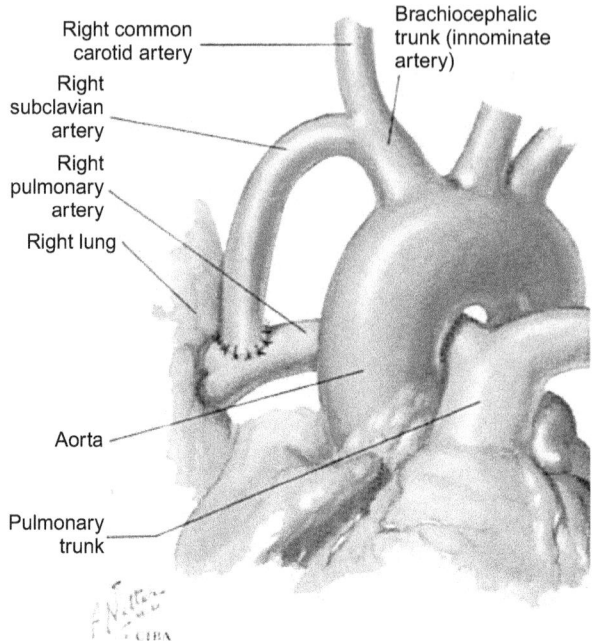

Right common carotid artery

Brachiocephalic trunk (innominate artery)

Right subclavian artery

Right pulmonary artery

Right lung

Aorta

Pulmonary trunk

FIGURE 14-1. Blalock-Taussig shunt to reduce severity of tetralogy of Fallot. Note that the right subclavian artery has been anastomosed to the right pulmonary artery. (From Van Mierop LH: Diseases—congenital anomalies. In Yonkman F, editor: **The heart,** Summit, NJ, 1969, Ciba-Geigy.)

Other Shunts

Glenn Shunt

A Glenn shunt connects the superior vena cava to the pulmonary artery (Figure 14-2). It is employed in infants at least 3 months old with tricuspid atresia or other complex congenital abnormalities (see Chapter 15) and normal pulmonary artery pressure. It does not generate a murmur. A Glenn shunt is often used as a prelude to a Fontan procedure (see Chapter 15), which is usually not done until after 2 years of age.

Potts Shunt

The Potts shunt is a direct anastomosis between the descending aorta and the left pulmonary artery. It was used in some children with tetralogy of Fallot in the early days of cardiac surgery, but has proved difficult to control and remove. Children with a Potts shunt, which is usually large, often develop congestive heart failure soon after the procedure and eventually develop pulmonary vascular disease. A Potts shunt generates a continuous murmur over the left posterior chest in children with low pulmonary vascular resistance. If pulmonary vascular resistance is high, the murmur is only systolic.

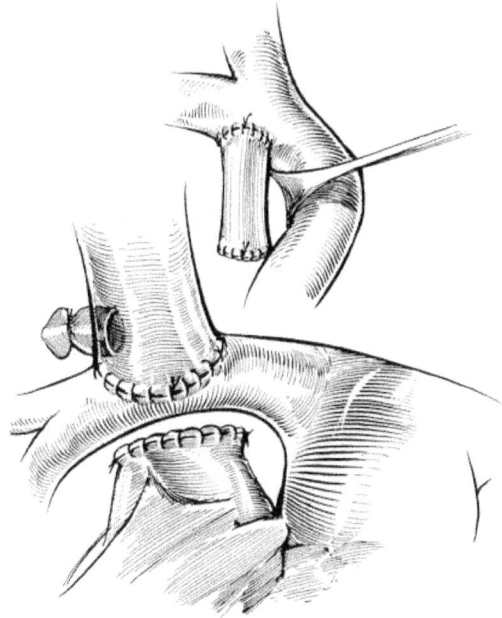

FIGURE 14-2. Bidirectional Glenn shunt showing the superior vena cava–right pulmonary anastomosis. (From Castañeda AR, Jonas RA, Mayer JE Jr et al: Single ventricle tricuspid atresia. In **Cardiac surgery of the neonate and infant,** Philadelphia, 1994, WB Saunders.)

Waterston Shunt

A Waterston shunt creates an anastomosis between the ascending aorta and the right pulmonary artery. The Waterston shunt has been used for some cases of tetralogy of Fallot but, like the Potts shunt, is complicated by congestive heart failure and the possibility of pulmonary vascular disease. A well-functioning Waterston shunt produces a continuous murmur, which is loudest at the upper right sternal border. The Potts and Waterston shunts are not widely employed today. A Blalock-Taussig or a controlled Gore-Tex central shunt is preferred.

PROSTHETIC VALVES

Prosthetic valves are used in children only as a last resort, and less than 10% of cases of congenital heart disease in children are treated with a prosthetic valve. Besides the rare outright failure, these valves can cause the destruction of red blood cells (hemolysis) as well as blood clots that may result in a stroke. Uneven blood flow through them permits pockets of blood to pool and coagulate. To prevent clotting, children with prosthetic valves must be given anticoagulants for their entire lives. Valves from humans (homografts) and pigs (porcine heterografts) do not require anticoagulation therapy but they commonly fail, usually because of calcification and occasionally infection.

The most common type of prosthetic valve is that used in a conduit repair (see Chapter 15). The second most common is the prosthetic aortic valve employed to relieve congenital aortic stenosis. The aortic valve is usually not replaced with a prosthetic valve until a second operation is performed, after a first attempt to repair the defective valve has failed. The Ross procedure, in which the patient's own pulmonary valve is used as an aortic autograft, is currently used as an alternative for surgical treatment of aortic valve disease.

The mechanical prosthetic valve most often used in children is the St. Jude bileaflet valve. The Bjork-Shiley tilting disk valve, once widely employed, is no longer manufactured. Surgeons also use the porcine (Hancock) heterograft. The heart sounds and murmurs made by prosthetic valves should be carefully recorded, because a change in these sounds suggests valve malfunction.

Bjork-Shiley Tilting Disk Valve

A Bjork-Shiley tilting disk valve is made of metal and other nonbiologic materials. It was taken off the market in 1986 because it may have a propensity to fail. Children with this valve require lifelong anticoagulation therapy.

In the aortic position, the opening sound is not usually audible. The closing sound is distinct, clicking, and high-pitched. Commonly the valve generates a grade II midsystolic ejection murmur, which is loudest in the aortic area. Rarely, there is a very faint (grade I) diastolic murmur, indicating very slight aortic regurgitation in a valve that is otherwise functioning well. If the valve begins to thrombose, the closing sound is audible, but a grade II to III diastolic murmur will develop, indicative of valve malfunction and aortic insufficiency.

St. Jude Bileaflet Valve

The St. Jude bileaflet valve, introduced in 1977, is a prosthetic valve in common use. It is made from pyrolytic carbon, a substance with very good tissue compatibility and a low tendency to cause thrombosis. Nevertheless, children with this valve require lifelong anticoagulation therapy.

The opening sound is generally not audible. When the valve is in the aortic position, there is usually a grade II early systolic to mid-systolic ejection murmur, best heard in the aortic area. The closing sound is distinct, clicking, and high-pitched. Loss of the closing sound is abnormal, a result of thrombosis, and may be accompanied by a grade III diastolic murmur indicating valve malfunction and aortic insufficiency.

Porcine (Hancock) Heterograft

The heterograft is a valve removed from the heart of a pig and preserved in glutaraldehyde. After the valve has been implanted, no anticoagulation is necessary.

The normal opening sound of a heterograft valve in the aortic position is not audible. The closing sound is high-pitched and discrete, audible in the aortic and pulmonic areas. It occupies the same position as A_2, and its relationship to P_2 is maintained. If the leaflets of the heterograft stenose and calcify, a loud ejection murmur develops. Aortic regurgitation generates a blowing diastolic murmur.

New Frontiers in Prosthetic Valve Design

To bring advanced technology to bear on the design of heart valves, a computer model of the flow of blood through the heart was used in the development of new prosthetic valves, now being patented and tested. The designers of the new valves claim that until now, the process of designing heart valves has not been especially rational or scientific.

The computer model produces diagrams that can be put together to make dramatic motion pictures of a two-dimensional but highly recognizable beating heart (Figure 14-3). Hundreds of dots, representing particles of blood, stream through the valve, stretching the elastic walls of the heart and creating whirling vortices. The purpose of the model is to portray the blood as discrete points, each with a speed and pressure affecting its neighbors in a way that can be calculated using physics equations. These thousands or millions of calculations must be repeated over and over again. To produce a realistic flow model of the heart, the flexibility and elasticity of the heart walls must be taken into account.

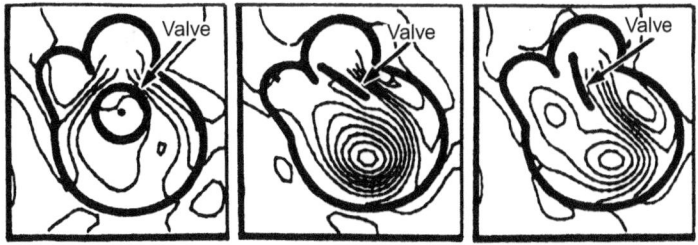

FIGURE 14-3. Computer model of blood flow through artificial valves: A ball in a cage **(left)** or a pivoting disk **(center).** The computer model indicates that the flow pattern is closest to normal when the disk shape is curved **(right).** (From McQueen DM, Peskin CS, Yellin EL: Fluid dynamics of the mitral valve: physiological aspects of a mathematical model, **Am J Physiol** 242:H1095-H1110, 1982.)

Instead of flowing over a rigid surface, as air flows over an airplane wing, blood deforms the heart surface, making the flow computation quite complex.

In Figure 14-3, computer images of blood flow through three types of artificial valves—a ball in cage, a pivoting disk valve, and a pivoting disk valve with a curved disk—are illustrated. The computer model indicates that the curved disk works best.

EVALUATION OF THE POSTOPERATIVE PATIENT

In the evaluation of a postoperative patient for whom there is no history, the type of procedure performed must be determined. A semihorizontal scar (a thoracotomy scar) on the side of the chest usually results from a shunt or repair of patent ductus arteriosus or coarctation of the aorta. If the child is cyanotic, the procedure was most likely a shunt, such as the Blalock-Taussig procedure. If there is a vertical midline scar, running from the top to bottom of the sternum (a median sternotomy scar), a definitive repair of the cardiac lesion was probably performed.

The interpretation of murmurs and sounds is different for the postoperative patient, and the examiner should not attempt to evaluate a postoperative patient as though he or she were an untouched preoperative one. For example, murmurs generated by a prosthetic valve may sound like valvular stenosis but may be compatible with a normally functioning artificial valve. A loud P_2, which might indicate pulmonary hypertension in a preoperative patient, is a normal finding if produced by a prosthetic valve. Also, particular sounds are associated with particular repairs. For example, a murmur of pulmonary regurgitation is expected in patients after correction of tetralogy of Fallot.

Some operations are curative. For example, a child may have a normal life span after correction of an atrial septal defect, ventricular septal defect, or patent ductus arteriosus. In such patients, no murmurs, or only innocent-sounding murmurs, are likely to be heard. In contrast, prosthetic valves may require replacement as the child grows. Likewise, the small conduit used to repair a truncus arteriosus in an infant may restrict flow as the child grows, and replacement with a larger conduit may be necessary. This must be explained to parents and reinforced at postoperative examinations.

BIBLIOGRAPHY

Doyle TP, Kavanaugh-McHugh A, Graham TP: Tetralogy of Fallot and pulmonary atresia with ventricular septal defect. In Moller JH, Hoffman JI, editors: **Pediatric cardiovascular medicine,** Philadelphia, 2000, Churchill Livingston.
Gleick J: Computers attack heart disease, **The New York Times,** Aug 5, 1986, p C1.
McQueen DM, Peskin CS, Yellin EL: Fluid dynamics of the mitral valve: physiological aspects of a mathematical model, **Am J Physiol** 242:H1095-H1110,

1982.

Syamsundar-Rao P: Tricuspid atresia. In Moller JH, Hoffman JI, editors: **Pediatric cardiovascular medicine,** Philadelphia, 2000, Churchill Livingston.

Tilkian AG, Conover MB: **Understanding heart sounds and murmurs,** ed 3, Philadelphia, 2001, WB Saunders.

Chapter 15

Complex Anomalies

Today most heart disease in children is congenital. Often several related cardiac lesions occur, rather than a single abnormality. Consequently, the differential diagnosis may involve deciding how many different murmurs (and lesions) are present.

This chapter describes some of the more important complex anomalies.

TETRALOGY OF FALLOT

Tetralogy of Fallot (Figure 15-1), first described in 1888, is composed of the following four abnormalities:

1. Ventricular septal defect
2. Pulmonic outflow obstruction
3. Aorta overriding right and left ventricles (i.e., biventricular aorta)
4. Right ventricular hypertrophy

Origin of the Murmur of Tetralogy of Fallot

In severe cases, pulmonic flow obstruction, from either pulmonic valve stenosis or, more commonly, infundibular stenosis, causes blood to be shunted from right to left through the ventricular septal defect and the overriding aorta.

In children with mild tetralogy of Fallot, who may not be cyanotic, the initial murmur often results from the left-to-right shunt through the ventricular septal defect. As the pulmonic stenosis becomes more severe, the murmur of pulmonic stenosis becomes increasingly audible. Eventually, the ventricular septal defect murmur from the left-to-right shunt disappears, and the resulting murmur is determined solely by the severity of pulmonic flow obstruction. In children with the most severe cases, who are the most cyanotic, there is little or no murmur, because most of the blood is shunted into the aorta through the septal defect, and very little flows through the pulmonic valve.

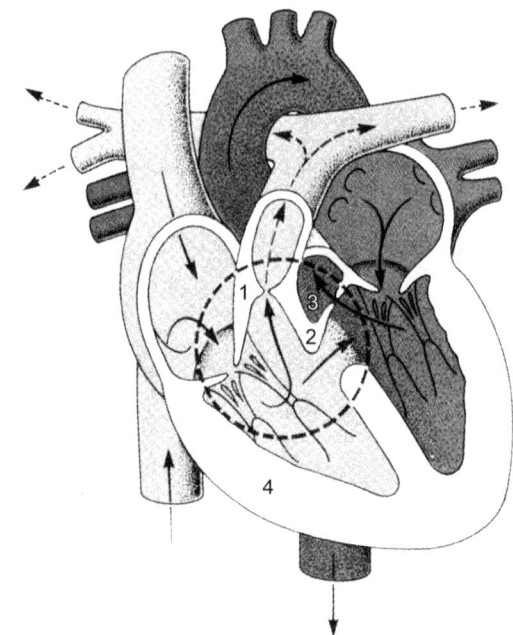

FIGURE 15-1. Tetralogy of Fallot, showing (1) pulmonic stenosis; (2) ventricular septal defect; (3) overriding aorta; and (4) right ventricular hypertrophy. Flow patterns are determined by the degree of pulmonic stenosis. (From Foster R, Hunsberger MM, Anderson JT: *Family-centered nursing care of children,* Philadelphia, 1990, WB Saunders.)

Nature of the Murmur of Tetralogy of Fallot

The murmur of tetralogy of Fallot is loudest along the left sternal border between the third and fourth interspaces. If a thrill can be palpated over this region, the murmur is at least grade III. The second heart sound tends to be single, because the pulmonic component is faint and hard to hear.

Differentiating Tetralogy of Fallot From Other Conditions
Pulmonic Stenosis With Intact Ventricular Septum

In patients with pulmonic stenosis and intact ventricular septum, the murmur is loudest in the most severe cases, whereas in patients with tetralogy of Fallot the murmur is softest in the most severe cases (Figure 15-2). The length of the murmur varies as well. In severe pulmonic stenosis, right ventricular systole is prolonged because of the outflow obstruction, and the murmur is relatively long. In severe tetralogy of Fallot, the right ventricle empties easily into the aorta and so the murmur is relatively short.

Prognosis

Usually some pulmonic insufficiency is present and is generally well tolerated after surgical repair of tetralogy of Fallot. Children are no longer cyanotic after repair, and the long-term prognosis is generally good.

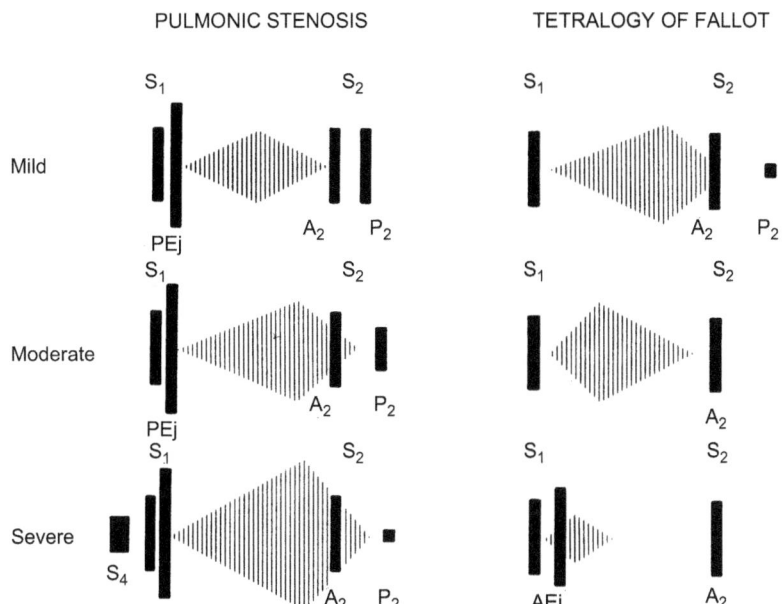

PULMONIC STENOSIS   TETRALOGY OF FALLOT

FIGURE 15-2. In valvular pulmonic stenosis with intact ventricular septum, right ventricular systolic ejection becomes progressively longer, with increasing obstruction to flow. As a result, the murmur becomes louder and longer, enveloping the aortic valve closure sound (A_2). The pulmonic valve closure sound (P_2) occurs later and splitting becomes wider but is more difficult to hear, because A_2 is lost in the murmur and P_2 becomes progressively fainter and lower pitched. As pulmonic diastolic pressure progressively decreases, isometric contraction shortens until the pulmonary valvular ejection sound fuses with the first heart sound (S_1). In severe pulmonic stenosis with concentric hypertrophy and decreasing right ventricular compliance, the fourth heart sound (S_4) appears.

In tetralogy of Fallot, with increasing obstruction at the pulmonic infundibular area, more and more right ventricular blood is shunted across a silent ventricular septal defect, and flow across the obstructed outflow tract decreases. Therefore, with increasing obstruction, the murmur becomes shorter, earlier, and fainter. P_2 is absent in severe tetralogy of Fallot. The large aortic root receives almost all cardiac output from both ventricular chambers, and the aorta dilates; this may be accompanied by an ejection click, which does not vary with respiration. *AEj*, Aortic ejection; *PEj*, pulmonary ejection; S_2, second heart sound. (From American Heart Association: *Examination of the heart. Part 4, Auscultation of the heart*, Dallas, 1990, American Heart Association.)

PERSISTENT TRUNCUS ARTERIOSUS COMMUNIS
Nature of the Defect

In persistent truncus arteriosus, a large single vessel arises from the heart, giving off the coronary arteries, the pulmonary arteries, and the aortic arch with its normal branches (Figure 15-3). The truncal valve is often tricuspid but may have two, four, or even six cusps. A large anterior ventricular septal defect is always present. Usually a short mainstem pulmonary artery divides into the left and right pulmonary arteries. In rare cases, the pulmonary arteries may arise separately from the trunk or may be absent, with pulmonary blood flow provided by bronchial collateral vessels arising from the descending aorta.

Clinical Features of Persistent Truncus Arteriosus

In the common form of truncus arteriosus, the clinical features are variable. The child may be very cyanotic, easily fatigued, and polycythemic, with clubbing of the fingers and shortness of breath on exertion. In an infant or very young child, cyanosis is often mild, and symptoms of heart failure predominate. These patients have shortness of breath, feeding difficulties, frequent respiratory infections, and failure to thrive.

Nature of the Murmur of Persistent Truncus Arteriosus

A child with persistent truncus arteriosus has a very active precordium. There is invariably a systolic murmur, often resulting from the ventricular septal defect but with elements of truncal valve stenosis and branch pulmonary artery stenosis, if these features are present. The murmur is loudest at the third or fourth intercostal space to the left of the sternum, sometimes associated with a thrill, often preceded by an ejection click. The first heart sound is normal. The second heart sound is quite loud and may be followed by a diastolic murmur caused by incompetence of the truncal valve.

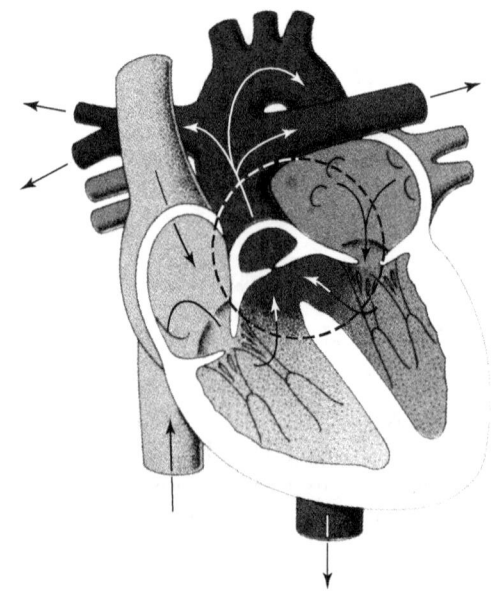

FIGURE 15-3. Truncus arteriosus. Blood flow is from both ventricles into a common great artery that overrides a ventricular septal defect. (From Daberkow E: Nursing strategies: altered cardiovascular function. In Foster RL, Hunsberger MM, Anderson JT, editors: *Family-centered nursing care of children,* Philadelphia, 1990, WB Saunders.)

Repair of Persistent Truncus Arteriosus

During the surgical repair of persistent truncus arteriosus (Figure 15-4), a conduit containing a valve is used to connect the right ventricle to the distal pulmonary arteries. The conduit may be a corrugated Dacron tube with a porcine valve or a fresh human aorta (aortic homograft).

The conduit makes abnormal sounds; its valve produces clicks. Systolic murmurs are usually present at three points: (1) the junction of the right ventricle and the conduit, (2) the valve, and (3) the junction of the conduit and the pulmonary artery. Sometimes the murmur of tricuspid regurgitation is also audible.

Prognosis

The conduit used in an infant is very small and requires replacement as the child grows. If aortic or truncal insufficiency exists, a newborn with truncus

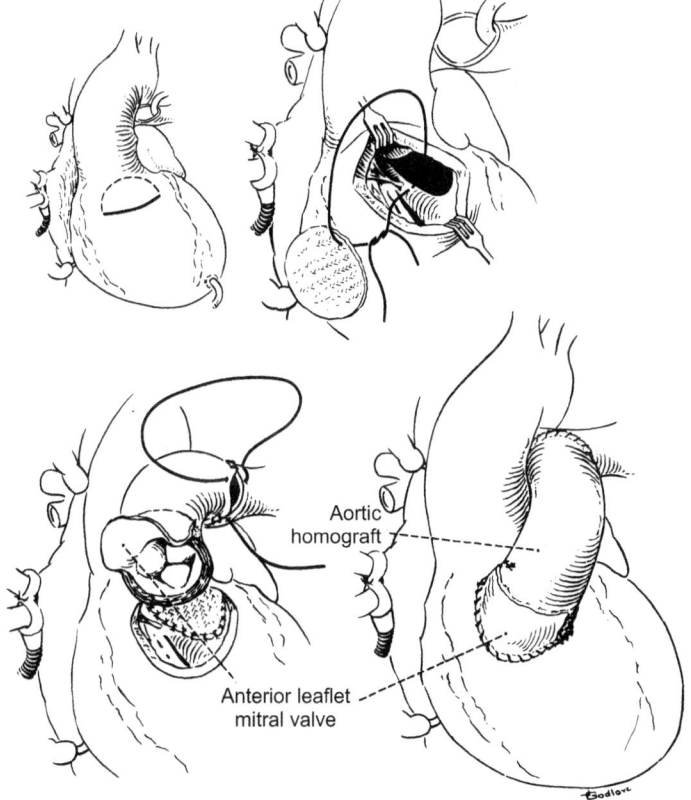

FIGURE 15-4. Steps in the repair of truncus arteriosus. The ventricular septal defect is repaired with a patch. An aortic homograft with its valve is used to connect the right ventricle to the previously disconnected pulmonary arteries. (From McGoon DC, Rastelli GC, Ongley PA: An operation for the correction of truncus arteriosus, *JAMA* 205:69, 1968.)

arteriosus may be so sick that the prognosis is quite poor. In older children, the prognosis depends on the exact anatomic abnormalities present and the degree of success in preventing undue elevation of pulmonary vascular resistance. If there are two separate pulmonary trunks coming off the side of the aorta, both repair and pulmonary artery banding (discussed later) are more difficult.

CARDIOVELOFACIAL SYNDROME

Many children with conotruncal lesions have the cardiovelofacial syndrome. Previously called the **DiGeorge syndrome,** the condition is also called **CATCH-22** (cardiac defects, abnormal facies, thymic hypoplasia, cleft palate, hypocalcemia, deletions in chromosome 22). Besides heart disease, children with this syndrome are deaf and have palatal abnormalities, learning disabilities, and emotional problems, with 10% to 15% developing schizophrenia during adolescence (Table 15-1).

TABLE 15–1. Noncardiac Features of CATCH-22 Syndrome

Minor Anomalies
Prominent nose with squared nasal root, malar flatness
Nasal dimple
Narrow palpebral fissures
Retruded mandible
Ear anomalies
Slender hands and fingers
Tortuous retinal vessels

Oral
Cleft palate (overt or submucous)
Velopharyngeal insufficiency
Pharyngoesophageal dysmotility, feeding problems

Immunologic
Absent thymus
T lymphocyte deficiencies
Low immunoglobulin levels

Endocrine
Hypoparathyroidism
Hypocalcemia
Short stature

Neurologic/Psychiatric
Speech disorder
Language delay and mental retardation
Sensorineural hearing loss
Attention deficit hyperactivity disorder
Bipolar disorder
Schizophrenia
Neural tube defects

From Johnson MC, Strauss AW: Genetic control in pediatric cardiovascular medicine. In Moller JH, Hoffman JI, editors: **Pediatric cardiovascular medicine,** Philadelphia, 2000, Churchill Livingston.

Fluorescence in situ hybridization (FISH) probes have shown chromosome 22q11 deletions in 75% to 90% of patients with CATCH-22. These deletions are also common in some conotruncal and aortic arch abnormalities. CATCH-22 may be one of the most common human deletion syndromes, with an estimated prevalence of 1:4000 to 1:9700. A single gene abnormality may be responsible, causing a neural crest defect in the embryologic third and fourth pharyngeal pouches.

Table 15-2 lists the prevalence of CATCH-22 deletions in conotruncal and arotic arch defects.

The caregiver should be aware of the noncardiac abnormalities in CATCH-22. Some children may have severe hypocalcemia and seizures, whereas others may have latent hypoparathyroidism with sudden, unexplained death. Therefore, calcium abnormalities should be monitored and aggressively treated in these children. Care of these children can be complicated, because failure to thrive may arise not only from uncorrected cardiac conditions, but also from feeding problems and other causes inherent in the syndrome.

ENDOCARDIAL CUSHION DEFECTS

Endocardial cushion defects result from a developmental abnormality of the atrioventricular endocardial cushions. These bulbous masses in the embryonic heart eventually form parts of the septum dividing the left and right sides of the heart and are also major contributors to the mitral and tricuspid valves (Figure 15-5).

Endocardial cushion defects are usually classified as complete or incomplete. In the complete defects, there is no separation of the mitral and tricuspid valve rings. In the incomplete defects, there are two separate valve rings, and the ostium primum atrial septal defect, which is the chief manifestation of the condition, may not be recognized until later in childhood.

TABLE 15–2. Prevalence of CATCH-22 Deletions in Conotrucal and Aortic Arch Defects

Defect	Prevalence (%)
Tetralogy of Fallot (TOF)	8
TOF/Pulmonary atresia	28
Absent pulmonic valve	64
Complete transposition	8
Interrupted aortic arch	40
Truncus arteriosus	10
Double outlet right ventricle	0
Origin of branch of pulmonary artery from aorta	67

Modified from Johnson MC, Strauss AW: Genetic control in pediatric cardiovascular medicine. In Moller JH, Hoffman JI, editors: **Pediatric cardiovascular medicine,** Philadelphia, 2000, Churchill Livingstone.

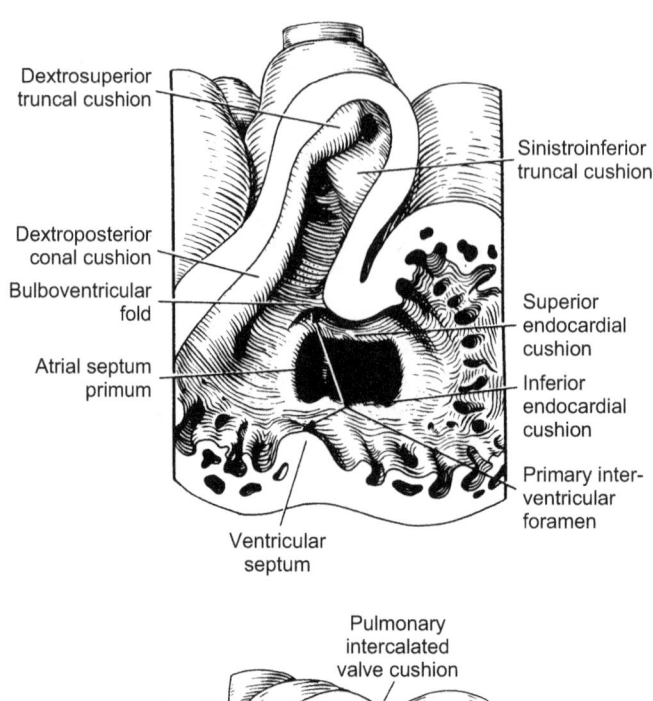

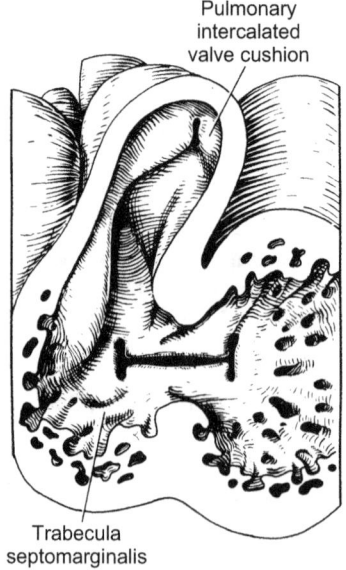

FIGURE 15-5. Schematic frontal section through the heart of two embryos. The endocardial cushions are bulbous masses or swellings that eventually form parts of the septum dividing the right and left sides of the heart. The endocardial cushions also make major contributions to the mitral and tricuspid valves. (From Van Mierop LHS, Alley RD, Kausel HW et al: The anatomy and embryology of endocardial cushion defects, *J Thorac Cardiovasc Surg* 43:71, 1962.)

Complete Endocardial Cushion Defect

Anatomic Anomalies

The most common complete endocardial cushion defect is the **persistent atrioventricular canal,** consisting of the following abnormalities (Figure 15-6):

1. A large, low atrial defect lies directly over the common atrioventricular valve ring, without a lower rim, and is contiguous with a posterosuperior ventricular septal defect.
2. A large cleft is present in the anterior leaflet of the mitral valve and in the septal leaflet of the tricuspid valve, so that the common anterior and posterior atrioventricular valve cusps serve both ventricles.
3. There is fusion of the adjoining mitral and tricuspid leaflets to form a butterfly-shaped single orifice.
4. The chordae tendineae are attached in part to the papillary muscles and in part to the top of the septum.

Clinical Features

Symptoms of persistent atrioventricular canal appear very early in life, with congestive heart failure usually present before 6 months of age. These children have poor weight gain, recurrent respiratory infections, and become dusky with feeding, crying, or exertion. In addition, persistent atrioventricular canal is very often associated with Down syndrome (in some studies, 35% to 40% of cases of Down syndrome are found in patients with this chromosomal abnormality); the signs of Down syndrome (see Chapter 3) should suggest the diagnosis of persistent atrioventricular canal.

Nature of the Heart Sounds and Murmurs in Persistent Atrioventricular Canal

The physical findings associated with persistent atrioventricular canal are dominated by the large shunt through the atrial and ventricular septal defects. The murmur of mitral regurgitation radiates to the left sternal edge and sometimes to the right anterior chest. A middiastolic tricuspid flow murmur may also occur. There is fixed splitting of the second heart sound and a prominent P_2 as well as a prominent right ventricular impulse.

Incomplete Endocardial Cushion Defect

Anatomic Anomalies

The incomplete (partial) endocardial cushion defect has the following characteristics (see Figure 15-6):

1. A large, low atrial septal defect (ostium primum atrial septal defect)
2. A cleft in the anterior leaflet of the mitral valve, which may result in

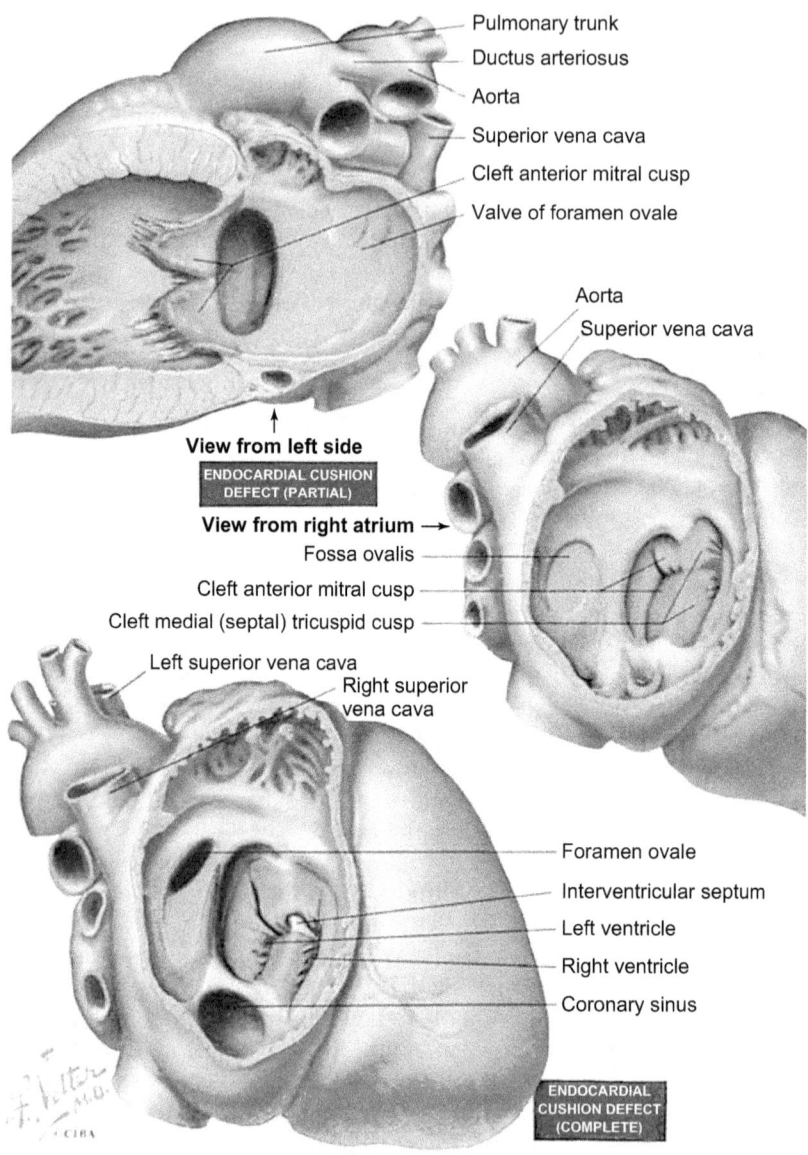

Pulmonary trunk
Ductus arteriosus
Aorta
Superior vena cava
Cleft anterior mitral cusp
Valve of foramen ovale

Aorta
Superior vena cava

View from left side
ENDOCARDIAL CUSHION
DEFECT (PARTIAL)

View from right atrium →
Fossa ovalis
Cleft anterior mitral cusp
Cleft medial (septal) tricuspid cusp
Left superior vena cava
Right superior
vena cava

Foramen ovale
Interventricular septum
Left ventricle
Right ventricle
Coronary sinus

ENDOCARDIAL
CUSHION DEFECT
(COMPLETE)

FIGURE 15-6. Endocardial cushion defect. In complete endocardial cushion defect *(lower drawing)*, there is total failure of the endocardial cushions to fuse, and the atrioventricular ostia form a large single ostium called a *persistent atrioventricular canal*. In a partial endocardial cushion defect *(upper drawing)*, if the endocardial cushions fuse only centrally, there is a division of the atrioventricular canal into right and left ostia, but the mitral valve, and often the septal cusp of the tricuspid valve, are cleft. (From Van Mierop LH: Diseases—congenital anomalies. In Yonkman F, editor: *The heart,* Summit, NJ, 1969, Ciba-Geigy.)

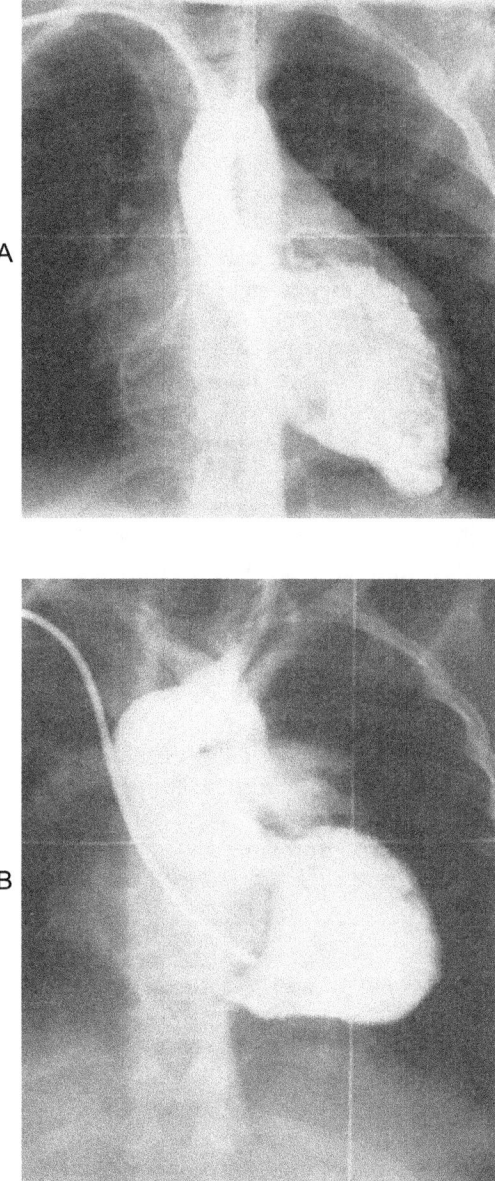

FIGURE 15-7. A, Normal left ventricular angiogram. Note the smooth walls with fine trabeculation (fishtail). **B,** Gooseneck deformity of the outflow region of the left ventricle in a patient with ostium primum defect. (From Nadas AS, Fyler DC: *Pediatric cardiology,* ed 3, Philadelphia, 1972, WB Saunders. Copyright AS Nadas.)

clinically apparent mitral insufficiency
3. Two separate valve rings
4. Intact ventricular septum (often but not always)
5. Abnormal location of mitral valve: displaced inferiorly, producing a characteristic gooseneck appearance on the angiogram (Figure 15-7)

Clinical Features

The clinical manifestations of partial endocardial cushion defect resemble those of atrial septal defect, although they often appear earlier and are more severe. Often, but not always, an incomplete AV canal defect is associated with growth retardation, fatigability, shortness of breath, and frequent respiratory infections. If mitral regurgitation is mild, there may be no symptoms for decades.

Nature of the Heart Sounds and Murmurs in Incomplete Endocardial Cushion Defect

Like an atrial septal defect, incomplete endocardial cushion defect produces a pulmonary ejection murmur and fixed splitting of the second sound. If pulmonary vascular resistance is high, P_2 may be loud, and there may be a loud S_3 at the apex. The systolic murmur of mitral insufficiency may also be heard, and its presence or absence is useful in distinguishing an atrial septal defect associated with endocardial cushion defect from an ostium secundum type of atrial septal defect. An ostium secundum type of atrial septal defect is rarely associated with mitral insufficiency. With a large shunt or marked mitral insufficiency, an early diastolic rumble at the lower left sternal border or apex is generated by the tricuspid or mitral valves (Figure 15-8) because of increased forward flow through them.

FIGURE 15-8. Phonocardiogram in a patient with an endocardial cushion defect. The upper tracing is obtained at the second left intercostal space, and the lower at the apex. Note the low-frequency, low-intensity systolic murmur at the second left intercostal space associated with the widely split second sound, third sound, and diastolic murmur. In the lower tracing, note the systolic murmur of mitral regurgitation and a diastolic flow murmur. *DM,* Diastolic murmur; *ECG,* electrocardiogram; *SM,* systolic murmur. (From Nadas AS, Fyler DC: *Pediatric cardiology,* ed 3, Philadelphia, 1972, WB Saunders. Copyright AS Nadas.)

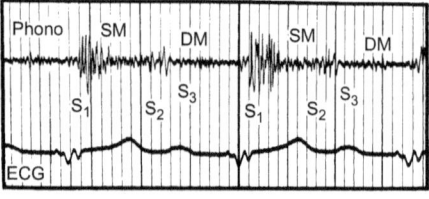
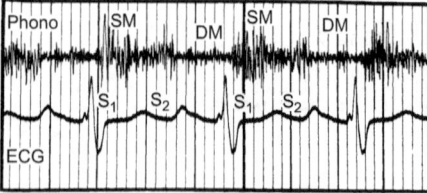

Prognosis

If there are severe mitral valve abnormalities, the mitral valve must often be replaced. After surgical repair, complete heart block may occur, and other rhythm abnormalities may develop with AV canal defects, in which the anatomy of the conduction system is abnormal.

TRICUSPID VALVE ANOMALIES

Among the congenital tricuspid valve abnormalities, only two have real clinical significance: tricuspid atresia and Ebstein's anomaly.

Tricuspid Atresia

Anatomic Anomalies

Tricuspid atresia, sometimes associated with transposition of the great vessels, is a common cause of severe cyanosis in a neonate. Tricuspid atresia has the following anatomic features (Figure 15-9):

1. A small dimple or an imperforate membrane where the opening of the tricuspid valve should be
2. A large, hypertrophied (thickened) left ventricle

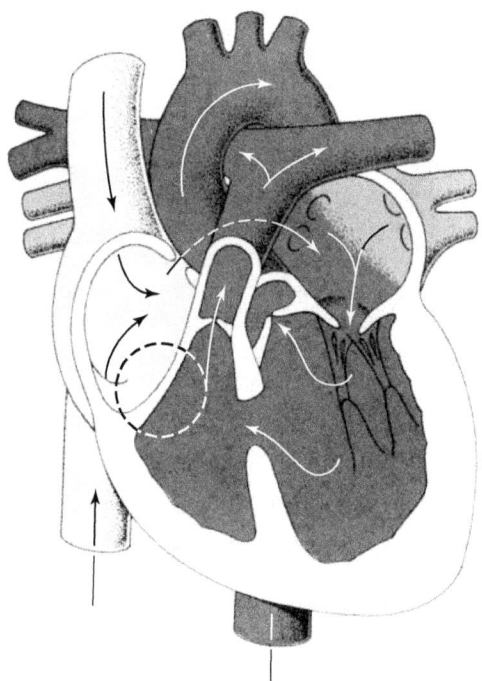

FIGURE 15-9. Tricuspid atresia, showing no communication between the right heart chambers. Blood is shunted through the atrial septal defect to the left atrium and through the ventricular septal defect to the pulmonary artery. (From Foster R, Hunsberger MM, Anderson JT: *Family-centered nursing care of children,* Philadelphia, 1990, WB Saunders.)

3. A very small or absent right ventricle
4. An interatrial communication
5. Possibly a ventricular septal defect
6. Usually severe pulmonary stenosis or pulmonary atresia if the great arteries are normally related

Clinical Features

Children with tricuspid atresia are very sick in early infancy. Blood flows from the right atrium to the left atrium, then to the left ventricle. If the great vessels are normal, blood flow to the lungs is via a ventricular septal defect to the right ventricle and pulmonary artery. Pulmonary blood flow is usually diminished, resulting in severe cyanosis, the dominant feature of tricuspid atresia. If transposition of the great vessels is present, pulmonary blood flow is increased and cyanosis is less prominent. With tricuspid atresia and transposition, the child is short of breath, easily fatigued, and has other symptoms suggestive of heart failure. There may be clubbing of the fingers in older children.

Nature of the Heart Sounds and Murmurs in Tricuspid Atresia

The apical heart sounds in tricuspid atresia are normal. The second heart sound has a diminished or absent P_2 because of the greatly reduced pulmonary blood flow. More than half of these patients have a harsh systolic murmur, loudest at the third intercostal space to the left of the sternum. This murmur is the result of the associated ventricular septal defect and pulmonic stenosis present in most patients with tricuspid atresia.

Surgical Treatment

The **Fontan procedure** is the best surgical method to correct tricuspid atresia. A connection is created between the right atrium and pulmonary artery, either by direct anastomosis or by insertion of a prosthetic conduit without a valve. The interatrial communication is then closed, allowing the right atrium to pump blood directly to the lungs, relieving cyanosis and reducing the burden on the single (left) ventricle. A modified Fontan procedure is shown in Figure 15-10. The Fontan procedure cannot be performed on an infant, however, and a shunt is usually necessary initially in children with severe cyanosis.

Prognosis

After the Fontan procedure, the immediate prognosis is good if pulmonary vascular resistance is normal. Because the procedure is relatively new, the long-term prognosis is still uncertain.

Ebstein's Anomaly

Anatomic Anomalies

In Ebstein's anomaly, a downward displacement of the tricuspid valve cusps occurs, except for the medial two thirds of the anterior cusp. The affected

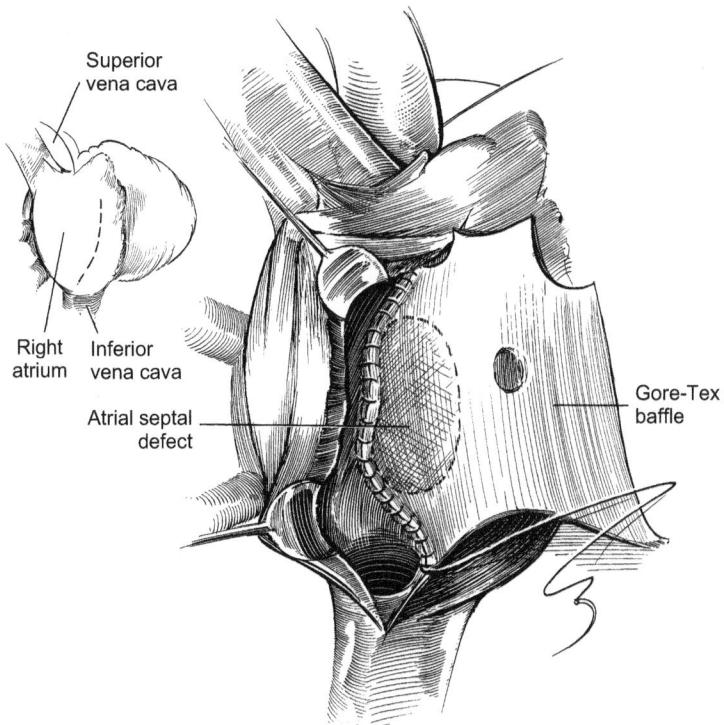

FIGURE 15-10. Modified Fontan (cavopulmonary isolation after end-to-side anastomosis of superior vena cava to the right pulmonary artery). Placement of baffle to convey inferior vena caval blood along the lateral wall of the right atrium to the superior vena caval orifice. A 4-mm fenestration is sometimes made on the medial aspect of the polytetrafluoroethylene baffle. (From Castañeda AR, Jonas RA, Mayer JE Jr et al: Single ventricle tricuspid atresia. In *Cardiac surgery of the neonate and infant,* Philadelphia, 1994, WB Saunders.)

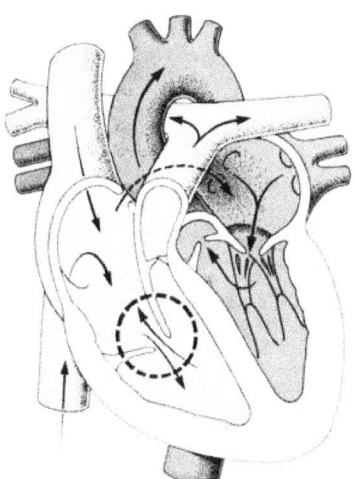

FIGURE 15-11. Ebstein's anomaly with the tricuspid valve significantly displaced downward in the right ventricle. Leakage occurs through the tricuspid valve back to the right atrium, and unoxygenated blood is shunted across the atrial septal defect (ASD) into the left atrium. (From Daberkow E: Nursing strategies: altered cardiovasacular function. In Foster RL, Hunsberger MM, Anderson JT, editors: **Family-centered nursing care of children,** Philadelphia, 1990, WB Saunders.)

cusps originate from the right ventricular wall rather than from the tricuspid annulus (Figure 15-11). The valve tissue is almost always redundant and wrinkled, and the chordae tendineae are poorly developed or absent.

Clinical Features

Patients with Ebstein's anomaly have considerable enlargement of the heart because of the large right atrium and atrialized right ventricle (Figure 15-12). They may be cyanotic, and their peripheral pulses are weak. The apical impulse is diffuse and poorly felt, and a precordial bulge and thrill are often present.

Nature of the Heart Sounds and Murmurs in Ebstein's Anomaly

The first heart sound is of normal intensity and may be split, the second (tricuspid) component being peculiarly loud. The second heart sound is normal. A loud, early diastolic third heart sound is present along the lower left sternal border, and a fourth heart sound may be audible. There may be a systolic murmur of tricuspid regurgitation, mild to moderate, along the left sternal border, and occasionally a diastolic murmur. The systolic murmur may sometimes have a scratchy quality, resembling a pericardial friction rub.

Prognosis

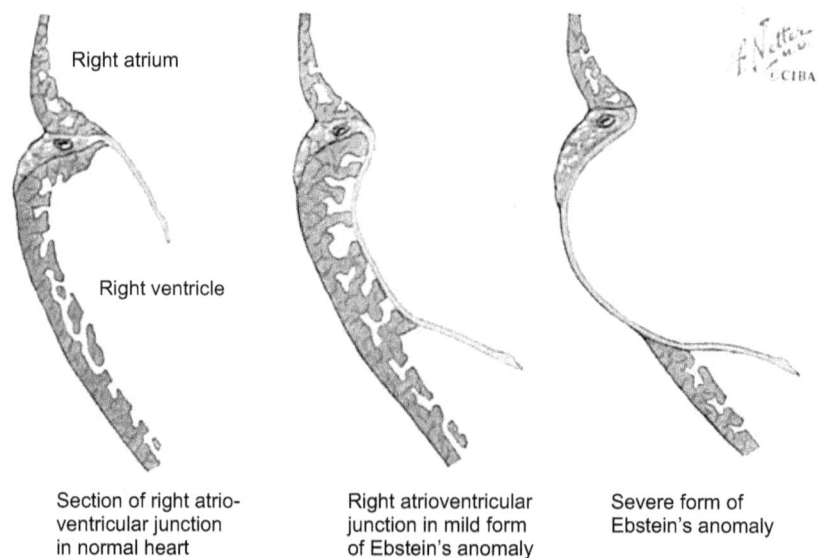

Right atrium

Right ventricle

| Section of right atrio-ventricular junction in normal heart | Right atrioventricular junction in mild form of Ebstein's anomaly | Severe form of Ebstein's anomaly |

FIGURE 15-12. Ebstein's anomaly. Note the downward displacement of the tricuspid valve. (From Van Mierop LH: Diseases—congenital anomalies. In Yonkman F, editor: *The heart*, Summit, NJ, 1969, Ciba-Geigy.)

Ebstein's anomaly is uncommon, and the prognosis is related to the severity of the lesion. In mild cases, no surgery is necessary. If the deformity is severe, the prognosis is poor.

TRANSPOSITION OF THE GREAT ARTERIES
Anatomic Anomalies

In simple complete transposition of the great arteries, a common malformation, the aorta arises anteriorly from the right ventricle, and the pulmonary trunk arises posteriorly from the left ventricle (Figure 15-13). The two arterial trunks are parallel to one another. In uncomplicated cases, the ventricles are normally formed, but the ventricular septum is intact in fewer than 50% of cases. Complete transposition occurs two to three times more often in boys than in girls.

Clinical Features

Transposition of the great vessels may cause heart failure in early infancy, especially in children who have a ventricular septal defect or patent ductus arteriosus. In children with an intact ventricular septum, severe cyanosis is the presenting symptom, and the infant is obviously cyanotic from birth. Cyanosis may become obvious later, within the first few days or weeks of

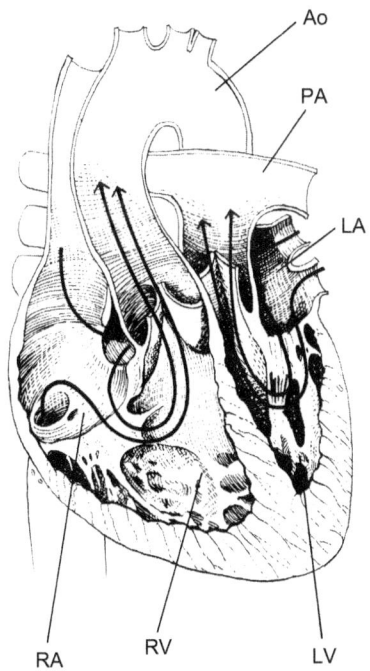

FIGURE 15-13. Complete transposition of the great arteries. Intercirculatory mixing occurs only at the atrial level. *Ao,* Aorta; *LA,* left atrium; *LV,* left ventricle; *PA,* pulmonary artery; *RA,* right atrium; *RV,* right ventricle. (From Braunwald E: *Heart disease,* ed 3, Philadelphia, 1988, WB Saunders.)

life, if another anomaly, such as ventricular septal defect, allows the pulmonary and systemic circulations to mix somewhat. If a large atrial or ventricular septal defect is present, the child may not become obviously cyanotic for months. The cyanosis increases when the child cries, but not so much as in tetralogy of Fallot.

In contrast to other forms of cyanotic heart disease, children with transposition have enlarged hearts, even shortly after birth. The antero-posterior diameter of the chest is increased, and a left precordial bulge may occur. The birth weight of a child with complete transposition of the great arteries is usually normal or increased, but feeding and weight gain are often poor. The child is short of breath and tends to breathe rapidly.

Nature of the Heart Sounds and Murmurs in Transposition of the Great Arteries

The first heart sound is normal or loud in transposition of the great arteries. Around the upper part of the sternum, the aortic component of the second heart sound (A_2) is loud because the aorta and aortic valve are close to the chest wall. The pulmonic component of the second heart sound (P_2) may be faint because the pulmonic valve is far posterior. A third heart sound is commonly audible. It is loudest at the lower left sternal border or just beneath it in deeply cyanotic children.

If there is no ventricular septal defect, there is often no murmur. If a ventricular septal defect is present, a systolic murmur occurs. Sometimes a diastolic mitral flow murmur can also be heard. If there is associated pulmonic stenosis, a thrill and a systolic murmur around the upper part of the sternum may result.

Prognosis

Most surgeons now perform an arterial switch procedure shortly after the child is born (Figure 15-14). Cardiologists anticipate that the long-term prognosis after the arterial switch procedure will be better than after the Mustard or Senning procedures, which redirect flow within the atria, leaving the right ventricle as the systemic ventricle. The Mustard and Senning operations often result in right ventricular dysfunction and arrhythmias.

CORRECTED TRANSPOSITION OF THE GREAT ARTERIES
Anatomic Anomalies

In corrected transposition of the great arteries, which affects boys two to three times as often as girls, the ascending aorta is in front of and parallel to the pulmonary trunk (Figure 15-15). The aorta arises anteriorly from the left-

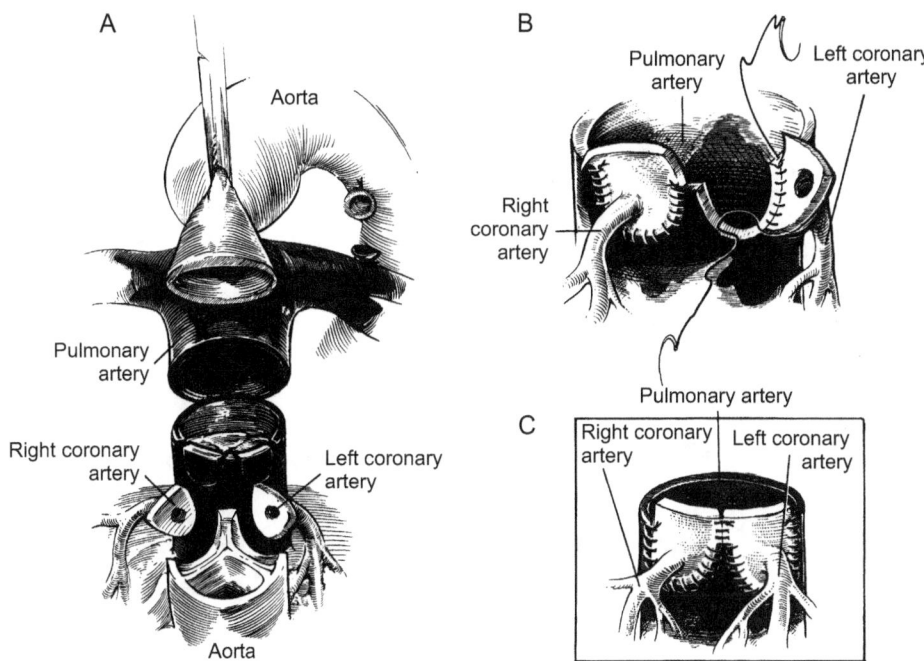

FIGURE 15-14. Method for translocating the coronary arteries in the arterial switch (Jatene) procedure. **A,** The aorta (anterior) and the pulmonary artery (posterior) have been transected, allowing visualization of the left and right coronary arteries. The coronaries have been excised from their respective sinuses, including a large flap (button) of arterial wall. Equivalent segments of the wall of the pulmonary artery (which will become neoaorta) are also removed. **B,** The aortocoronary buttons are sutured into the proximal neoaorta. With this technique all sutures are placed in the button of aortic wall, rather than directly on the coronary arteries. **C,** Completed anastomosis of the left and right coronary arteries to the neoaorta. (From Castañeda AR, Jonas RA, Mayer JE Jr et al: Single ventricle tricuspid atresia. In *Cardiac surgery of the neonate and infant,* Philadelphia, 1994, WB Saunders.)

sided ventricle, and the pulmonary trunk arises posteriorly from the right-sided ventricle—the reverse of a normal configuration. In addition, the right-sided ventricle is structurally like a normal left ventricle and has a mitral valve. The left-sided ventricle structurally resembles a right ventricle and has a tricuspid valve. The two atria are normal.

Unlike complete transposition, in corrected transposition the circulation is physiologically normal. The aorta receives arterial blood and the pulmonary artery receives venous blood. Problems occur because of other associated anomalies. The left-sided atrioventricular valve, structurally a tricuspid valve, is often malformed and incompetent because of Ebstein's anomaly. Also, there may be a ventricular septal defect or pulmonary stenosis or both, and the conduction system is anatomically abnormal.

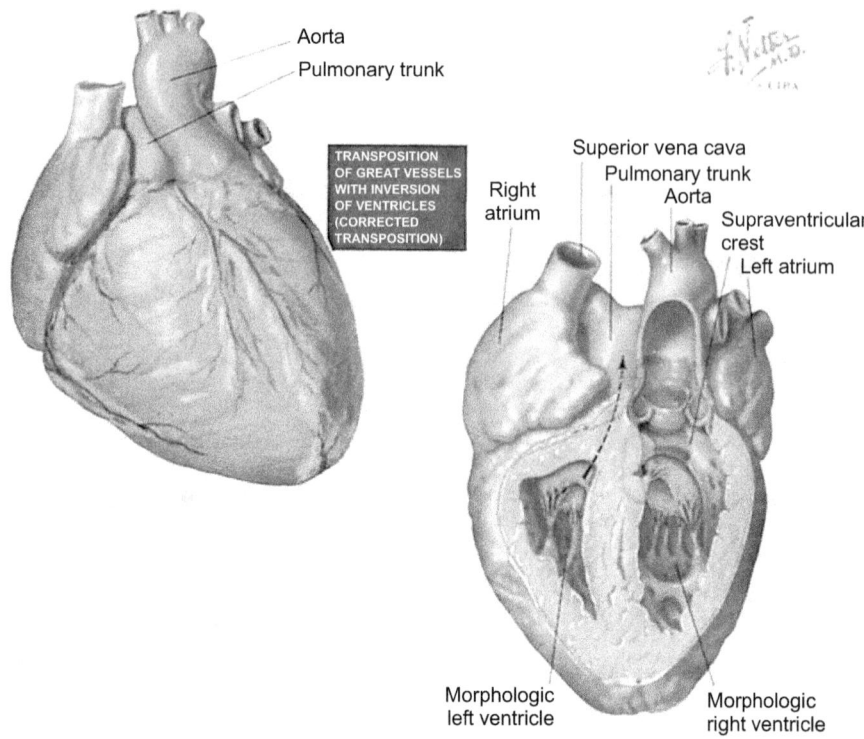

FIGURE 15-15. Corrected transposition of the great vessels. The ascending aorta is in front of and parallel to the pulmonary trunk. The aorta arises anteriorly from the left-sided ventricle (morphologically a right ventricle); the pulmonary trunk arises from the right-sided ventricle (morphologically a left ventricle). (From Van Mierop LH: Diseases—congenital anomalies. In Yonkman F, editor: *The heart,* Summit, NJ, 1969, Ciba-Geigy.)

Nature of the Heart Sounds and Murmurs in Corrected Transposition of the Great Arteries

The heart block and prolonged P-R interval often present in corrected transposition may cause the first heart sound to be soft (see Chapter 6). In cases in which complete heart block is present, the intensity of the first heart sound varies. The first component of the second heart sound (A_2) is loud and clear in the second left intercostal space (the pulmonic area) because the ascending aorta and aortic valve are anterior and on the left, rather than posterior and on the right, as in a normal child. The pulmonic component of the second heart sound (P_2) is damped because the pulmonary artery and pulmonic valve are posterior.

Half the time an apical systolic murmur results from left-sided tricuspid regurgitation. When pulmonic stenosis is present, there is a systolic murmur, loudest at the second intercostal space to the right of the sternum (the aortic area). (Remember that the pulmonary artery is on the right, rather than in its normal position on the left.) If the obstruction is subpulmonic, the murmur may be loudest in the third left intercostal space. If a ventricular septal defect exists, a holosystolic murmur in the third or fourth intercostal space to the left of the sternum occurs.

Prognosis

After surgical correction for associated defects, patients with L-transposition frequently have complete heart block and rhythm abnormalities, although these can also be seen in nonoperated patients. Associated ventricular septal defect, pulmonic stenosis, or left Ebstein's anomaly is usually the reason for surgery.

HYPOPLASTIC LEFT HEART SYNDROME
Anatomic Anomalies

Hypoplastic left heart syndrome (Figure 15-16) is a group of similar heart abnormalities with the following characteristics:

1. Underdevelopment of the left atrium and left ventricle, sometimes accompanied by endocardial fibroelastosis

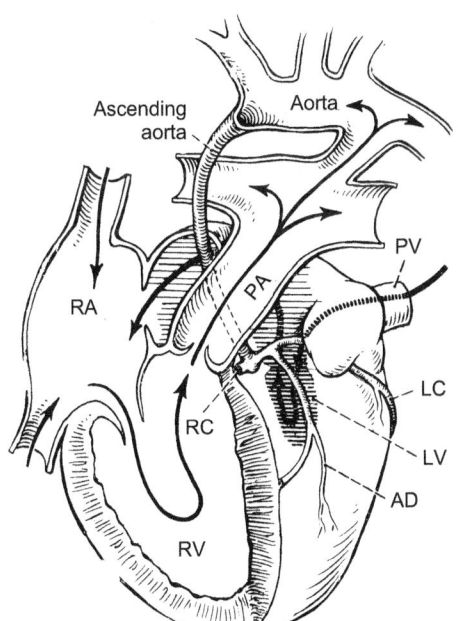

FIGURE 15-16. Hypoplastic left heart with aortic hypoplasia, aortic valve atresia, and a hypoplastic mitral valve and left ventricle. *AD,* Anterior descending coronary artery; *LC,* left coronary artery; *LV,* left ventricle; *PA,* pulmonary artery; *PV,* pulmonary vein; *RA,* right atrium; *RC,* right coronary artery; *RV,* right ventricle. (From Neufeld HN, Adams P, Edwards JE et al: Diagnosis of aortic atresia by retrograde aortography, *Circulation* 25:278, 1962.)

2. Atresia or stenosis of the aortic valve
3. Atresia or stenosis of the mitral valve
4. Hypoplasia (underdevelopment) of the ascending aorta

In addition, the muscular wall of the right ventricle is thickened and the chamber is dilated. The right ventricle pumps both systemic and pulmonary blood. Pulmonary venous blood passes through an open foramen ovale. Immediately after birth, the systemic circulation receives blood through a patent ductus arteriosus.

Clinical Features of Hypoplastic Left Heart Syndrome

Hypoplastic left heart syndrome, which occurs most commonly in boys, is one of the most common causes of neonatal death from congenital heart disease. Once the ductus arteriosus closes, the infant suddenly becomes critically ill and listless, with marked cyanosis. Brachial, carotid, and femoral pulses are barely palpable. A strong right ventricular impulse can be felt on palpation of the chest.

Nature of the Heart Sounds and Murmurs in Hypoplastic Left Heart Syndrome

Despite the gravity of the disease, the auscultatory findings in hypoplastic left heart syndrome are unimpressive. The aortic component of the second heart sound is absent, and the pulmonic component is loud. There is usually no murmur, although a soft midsystolic murmur may be produced by the flow of blood into the dilated pulmonary trunk. Tricuspid regurgitation may cause a loud holosystolic murmur. A summation gallop is often audible (see Chapter 8).

Prognosis

The prognosis is not good. A palliative operation, the Norwood procedure, can be performed (Figure 15-17), followed later by a Fontan procedure. In other cases, a heart transplant is performed, but donor availability limits this operation.

TOTAL ANOMALOUS PULMONARY VENOUS CONNECTION
Nature of the Defect

In total anomalous pulmonary venous connection, all pulmonary and systemic veins enter the right atrium. Remember that normally the systemic veins enter the right atrium, and the pulmonary veins enter the left atrium. The systemic circulation then receives partially oxygenated blood from a common pool, created by a right-to-left shunt through a patent foramen ovale or atrial septal defect (see Figure 8-6).

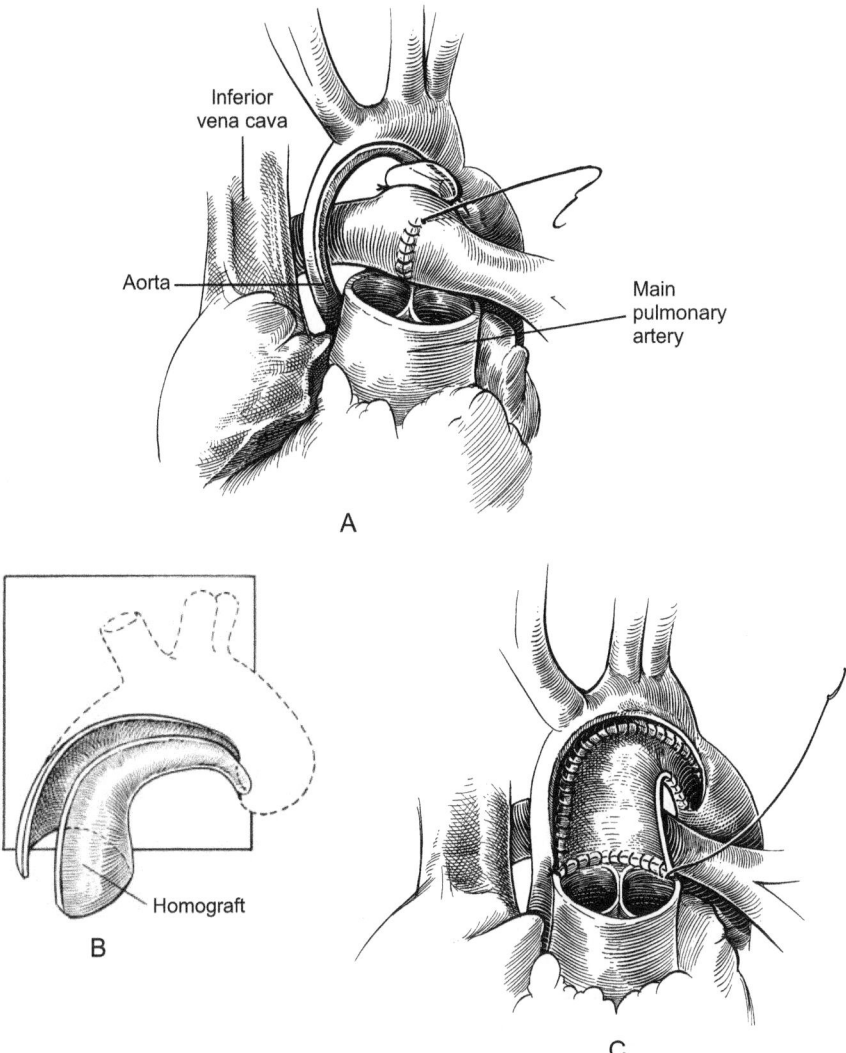

FIGURE 15-17. Current technique for first-stage palliation of the hypoplastic left heart syndrome. **A,** Incisions used for the procedure, incorporating a cuff of arterial wall allograft. The distal divided main pulmonary artery may be closed by direct suture or with a patch. **B,** Dimensions of the cuff of the arterial wall allograft. **C,** The arterial wall allograft is used to supplement the anastomosis between the proximal divided main pulmonary artery and the ascending aorta, aortic arch, and proximal descending aorta. (From Castañeda AR, Jonas RA, Mayer JE Jr et al: Single-ventricle tricuspid atresia. In *Cardiac surgery of the neonate and infant,* Philadelphia, 1994, WB Saunders.)

Continued

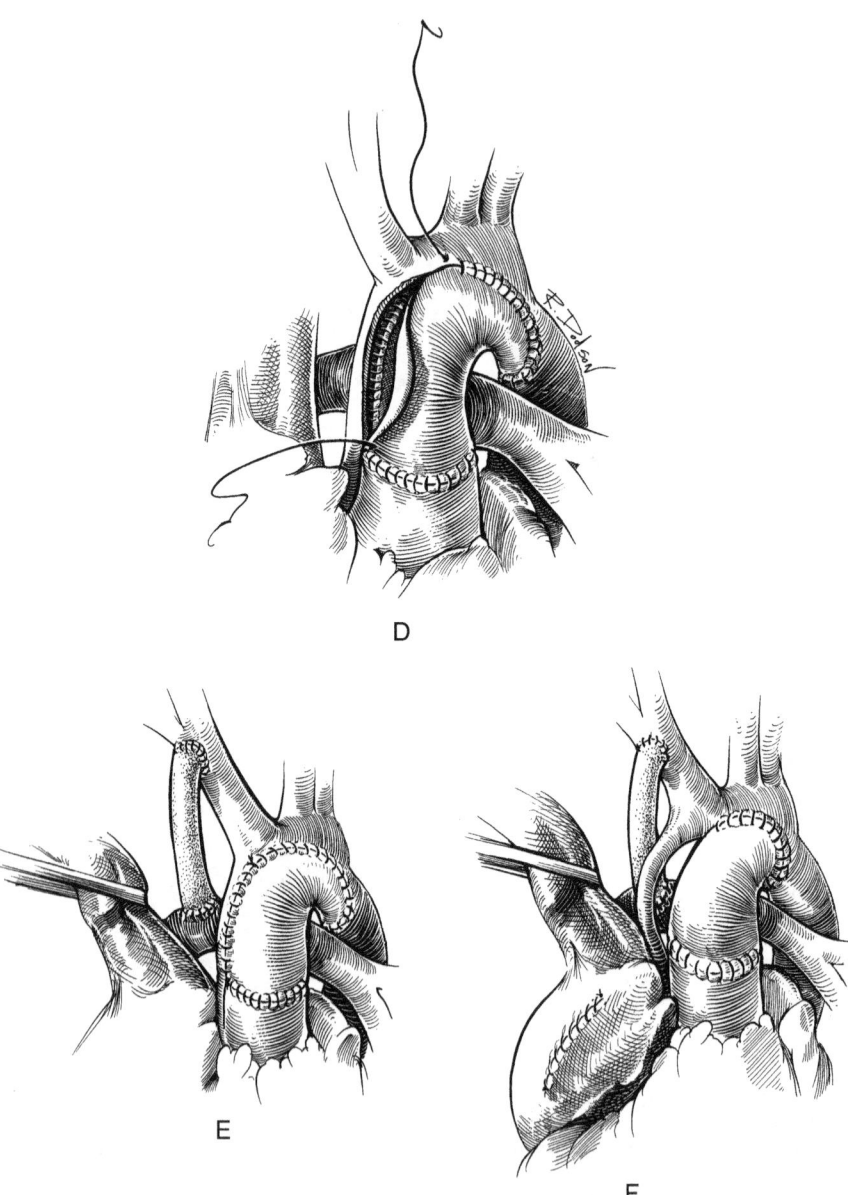

FIGURE 15-17, cont'd. D and **E,** The procedure is completed by an atrial septectomy and a 3.5-mm modified right Blalock shunt. **F,** When the ascending aorta is particularly small, an alternative procedure involves placement of a complete tube of arterial allograft. The tiny ascending aorta may be left in situ, as indicated, or implanted into the side of the neoaorta.

Clinical Features of Total Anomalous Pulmonary Venous Connection

When there is good pulmonary blood flow, the infant is only mildly cyanotic and short of breath, and the anomaly may be overlooked. However, with time cyanosis increases, and there is more shortness of breath. The child has recurring respiratory infections, feeding difficulties, and growth and development lag. There is usually a right ventricular heave. If the condition goes untreated, 90% of affected children die within a year. If there is obstruction within the anomalous venous channel, the child will die within the first few weeks of life if surgery is not performed.

Heart Sounds in Total Anomalous Pulmonary Venous Connection

The heart sounds in total anomalous pulmonary venous connection resemble those in atrial septal defect (Figure 15-18). The first heart sound is prominent and often followed by an ejection click. There may be a mid-systolic murmur in the second left intercostal space (pulmonary area). A wide, fixed splitting of the second heart sound occurs, and often P_2 is very loud, especially if pulmonary veins are obstructed. There may be third and fourth heart sounds. Half the cases have a diastolic tricuspid flow murmur at the lower left sternal border. If the anomalous connection is to the left innominate vein, there may be a venous hum in the pulmonary area (Figure

FIGURE 15-18. Phonocardio-gram of patient with total anomalous pulmonary venous connection. Note the systolic murmur *(SM)* and the four heart sounds. *4LIS,* Fourth left intercostal space. (From Nadas AS, Fyler DC: *Pediatric cardiology,* ed 3, Philadelphia, 1972, WB Saunders. Copyright AS Nadas.)

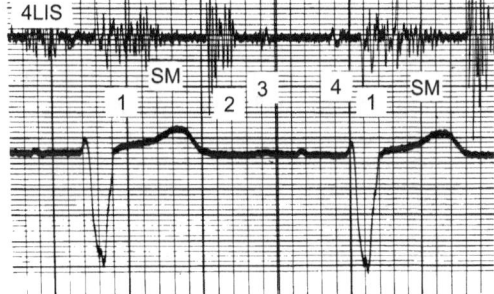

FIGURE 15-19. Continuous murmur in a patient with total anomalous pulmonary venous connection. *DM,* Diastolic murmur; *SM,* systolic murmur. (From Nadas AS, Fyler DC: *Pediatric cardiology,* ed 3, Philadelphia, 1972, WB Saunders. Copyright AS Nadas.)

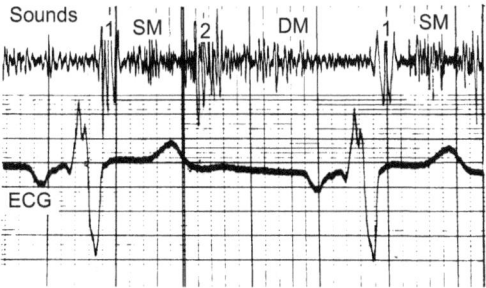

15-19). Unlike the innocent venous hum (see Chapter 11), the venous hum of total anomalous pulmonary venous connection is not altered by change in position or pressure on the neck veins. Often no characteristic murmur is present, making clinical recognition of this condition difficult.

Prognosis

Many of these infants are very sick. The outlook is often good if the child survives surgery. If the anomalous pulmonary venous connection is below the diaphragm, severe pulmonic obstruction occurs soon after birth, and surgery must be scheduled immediately on diagnosis.

DOUBLE OUTLET RIGHT VENTRICLE
Nature of the Defect

In double outlet right ventricle, the aorta is on the right; thus, the aorta and pulmonary artery both arise from the right ventricle. Four major types of double outlet right ventricle are shown in Figure 15-20. Pulmonic stenosis affects more than half of patients. A ventricular septal defect is always present.

Clinical Features of Double Outlet Right Ventricle

Cyanosis is absent or very mild in infants without pulmonic stenosis. If pulmonic stenosis is present, cyanosis becomes evident within the first year of life.

The child suffers recurrent respiratory infections and poor growth and development. Without surgery, an occasional patient reaches young adulthood, but most develop progressive pulmonary vascular obstruction and chronic congestive heart failure. Some cases of trisomy 18, with distinctive overlapping fingers, rocker bottom feet, and lax skin (see Figure 13-7), are associated with double outlet right ventricle. The precordium is bulging and overactive. Harrison's grooves may be present, indicating poor pulmonary compliance because of a large left-to-right shunt (Figure 3-6). A thrill of ventricular septal defect may be palpable in the third or fourth intercostal spaces at the left sternal edge.

Heart Sounds in Double Outlet Right Ventricle

The first heart sound is normal or soft because of a prolonged P-R interval (see Chapter 6). There may be a single second heart sound. In children with low pulmonary vascular resistance, a holosystolic murmur of ventricular septal defect is present, maximal in the third or fourth intercostal spaces at the left sternal edge. If pulmonary vascular resistance rises, pulmonary blood flow diminishes; the murmur of ventricular septal defect then softens and becomes

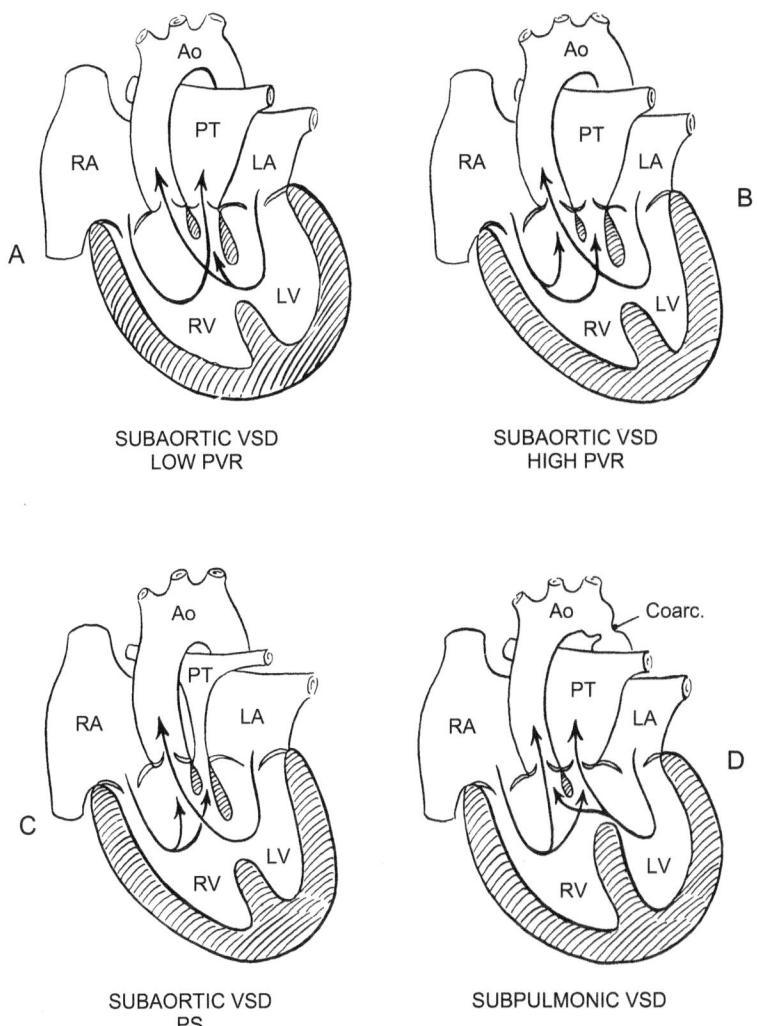

FIGURE 15-20. Four major clinical patterns of double outlet right ventricle. **A,** Subaortic ventricular septal defect *(VSD),* low pulmonary vascular resistance *(PVR),* and no pulmonic stenosis. **B,** Subaortic VSD with high pulmonary vascular resistance.
C, Subaortic VSD with pulmonic stenosis *(PS).* **D,** Subpulmonic VSD with variable pulmonary vascular resistance (Taussig-Bing anomaly). *Ao,* Aorta; *LA,* left atrium; *LV,* left ventricle; *PT,* pulmonary trunk; *RA,* right atrium; *RV,* right ventricle. (From Perloff JK: *The clinical recognition of congenital heart disease,* ed 4, Philadelphia, 1994, WB Saunders.)

decrescendo.

Pulmonary Artery Banding

In complex lesions with increased pulmonary flow, such as double outlet right ventricle, pulmonary arterial banding can be performed during the first year of life. The banding reduces pulmonary flow, thereby relieving the volume overload causing congestive heart failure. Banding also protects the pulmonary arterioles, and prevents them from developing pulmonary arteriopathy leading to irreversible pulmonary vascular disease.

Prognosis

Intracardiac repair of double outlet right ventricle is usually not performed in early infancy. The prognosis is worse than after repair of tetralogy of Fallot. Also, a mistake can be made in which double outlet right ventricle is confused with simple ventricular septal defect, whereupon the ventricular septal defect is closed with disastrous results.

ASPLENIA AND POLYSPLENIA

Severe congenital heart disease sometimes occurs in children with abnormalities of the spleen, either asplenia (absence of the spleen) or polysplenia (the presence of multiple small masses of splenic tissue). These children also have malposition of the heart, liver, stomach, and other sections of the gastrointestinal tract.

Asplenia

Anatomic Anomalies
Children with asplenia, mostly boys, have duplication or persistence of right-sided structures and the absence or displacement of left-sided structures. Specific abnormalities include the following:

1. An abnormally symmetrical liver (transverse liver) situated across both sides of the upper abdomen (Figure 15-21)
2. Displacement of the stomach to the right side of the abdomen
3. A left lung with three lobes instead of the normal two
4. Both atria structurally resemble a right atrium

Clinical Features
A child with asplenia is usually a very young male infant with severe cyanosis and a symmetric liver. The cardiovascular anomalies are listed in Table 15-3. **Howell-Jolly bodies** in the peripheral blood smear are a characteristic finding (Figure 15-22). One third of asplenic infants die within

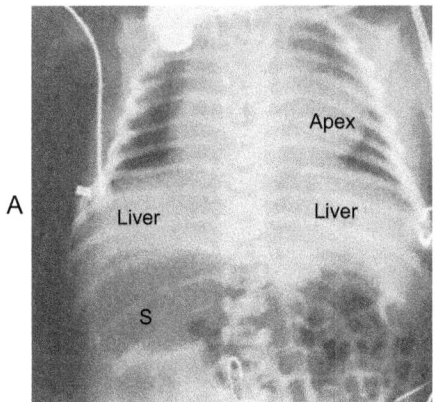
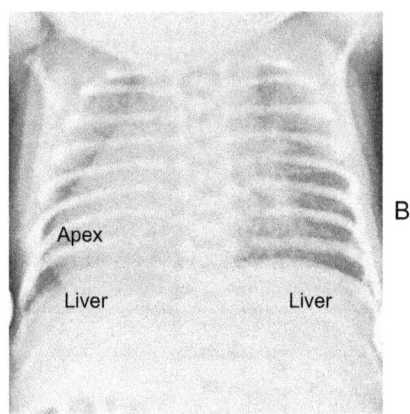

FIGURE 15-21. A, Chest x-ray film from an asplenic male neonate. The most important radiologic feature is the transverse liver. The stomach *(S)* is on the right. The heart is relatively central, but the base-to-apex axis points to the left. **B,** Chest x-ray film from an asplenic male neonate. The liver is transverse. The major portion of the cardiac silhouette is to the right of the midline. The ground-glass appearance of the lung fields is caused by obstructive total anomalous pulmonary venous connection. (From Perloff JK: *The clinical recognition of congenital heart disease,* ed 4, Philadelphia, 1994, WB Saunders.)

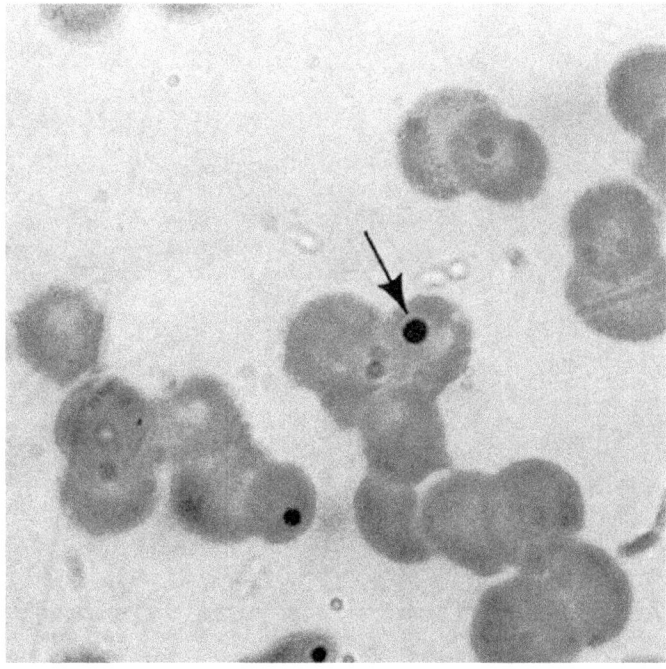

FIGURE 15-22. Peripheral blood smear showing Howell-Jolly bodies *(arrow)* in a patient with asplenia. (From Perloff JK: *The clinical recognition of congenital heart disease,* ed 4, Philadelphia, 1994, WB Saunders.)

a week of birth; only 15% survive a year. Sudden, overwhelming bacterial infection is a constant hazard.

Asplenic infants are almost always cyanotic. Physical examination reveals a right-sided heart through percussion, and the liver edge is palpable across the entire upper abdomen.

Polysplenia

TABLE 15–3. Cardiovascular Abnormalities in Asplenia and Polysplenia Syndromes

	Asplenia (%)	Polysplenia (%)
Cardiac Position		
Dextrocardia	41	42
Levocardia	59	58
Great Arteries		
Normal relations	19	84
Transposition	72	8
Double outlet RV	9	8
Pulmonic Valve		
Normal	22	58
Pulmonary stenosis	34	33
Pulmonary atresia	44	9
Great Veins		
Normal	16	50
TAPVC	72	0
PAPVC	6	42
Absent infrahepatic suprarenal IVC	0	84
Bilateral SVC	53	33
Atrial Septum		
Intact	0	16
Primum ASD	100	42
Secundum ASD	66	26
Single atrium	0	16
Atrioventricular Valves		
Two	13	50
Single or common	87	16
Ventricular Septum		
Intact	6	25
Single ventricle	44	8
Atrioventricular canal	50	33
Other VSD	3	33
Coronary Arteries		
Single	19	0
Coronary Sinus		
Absence	85	42

From Rose V, Izukawa T, Moes CAF: Syndromes of asplenia and polysplenia. A review of cardiac and noncardiac malformations in 60 cases with special references to diagnosis and prognosis, **Br Med J** 37:840, 1975.
ASD, Atrial septal defect; **IVC,** inferior vena cava; **PAPVC,** partial anomalous pulmonary venous connection; **RV,** right ventricles; **SVC,** superior vena cava; **TAPVC,** total anomalous pulmonary venous connection; **VSD,** ventricular septal defect.

Anatomic Anomalies

In children with polysplenia, which is most common in girls, the liver is abnormally symmetric in a quarter of cases, and the stomach is on the right in two thirds of cases. The right lung has two lobes instead of the normal three.

The cardiovascular malformations are listed in Table 15-3.

Clinical Features

Birth weight is usually normal, and cyanosis is mild or absent. Intractable heart failure is the most common cause of death. A right-sided heart and transverse liver may be detected on physical examination. Until recently, one third of the children with this condition died within a month of birth and half died within 4 months. A quarter survived 5 years, and 10% were alive at midadolescence. Today, however, with increasingly sophisticated medical and surgical management, an increasing proportion of children with complex defects survive.

BIBLIOGRAPHY

Alley RD, Van Mierop LH: Diseases—congenital anomalies. In Yonkman F, editor: **The heart,** Summit, NJ, 1969, Ciba-Geigy.

de Leval M: Lessons from the arterial switch operation, **Lancet** 357:1814, 2001.

Freed MD: The pathology, pathophysiology, recognition, and treatment of congenital heart disease. In Fuster V, Alexander RW, O'Rourke RA, editors: **Hurst's the heart,** New York, 2001, McGraw-Hill.

Freedom RM: Congenitally corrected transposition of the great arteries. In Moller JH, Hoffman JI, editors: **Pediatric cardiovascular medicine,** Philadelphia, 2000, Churchill Livingston.

Friedman WF, Silverman N: Congenital heart disease in infancy and childhood. In Braunwald E, Zipes DP, Libby P, editors: **Heart disease,** ed 6, Philadelphia, 2001, WB Saunders.

Johnson MC, Strauss AW: Genetic control in pediatric cardiovascular medicine. In Moller JH, Hoffman JI, editors: **Pediatric cardiovascular medicine,** Philadelphia, 2000, Churchill Livingston.

Nadas A, Fyler DC: **Pediatric cardiology,** ed 3, Philadelphia, 1972, WB Saunders.

Perloff JK: **The clinical recognition of congenital heart disease,** ed 4, Philadelphia, 1994, WB Saunders.

Prêtre R, Tamisier D, Bonhoeffer P et al: Results of the arteria switch operation in neonates with transposed great arteries, **Lancet** 357:1826-1830, 2001.

Sidi D: Complete transpositon of the great arteries. In Moller JH, Hoffman JI, editors: **Pediatric cardiovascular medicine,** Philadelphia, 2000, Churchill Livingston.

Glossary

Abscess. A localized collection of pus in any part of the body.

Anastomosis. Establishing a surgical connection between two hollow organs (e.g., the anastomosis of two arteries).

Aneurysm. A ballooning of the wall of an artery or structure within the heart.

Annulus. Valve ring.

Anomaly. Abnormality.

Anoxic. Without oxygen.

Antecedent. That which comes before.

Anticonvulsant. Medication that prevents seizures.

Aorta. The large vessel arising from the left ventricle and distributing, by its branches, arterial blood to every part of the body.

Arrhythmia. Abnormal heart rhythm.

Ascites. A collection of fluid in the abdominal cavity.

Asystole. No heartbeat.

Ataxia. Incoordination of muscular action.

Ataxia, Friedreich's. A progressive familial disease occurring in childhood characterized by incoordination, absent deep reflexes, speech disturbance, jerky eye movements (nystagmus), and clubfoot.

Atherosclerosis. A clogging of the arteries by fatty deposits.

Atresia. Imperforation or closure of a normal opening or canal, such as atresia of the pulmonic valve.

Auscultation. Listening to the sounds of the body, usually with the aid of a stethoscope.

Axilla. Armpit.

Bigeminy. A premature ventricular contraction coupled with each normal heartbeat.

Bradycardia. Slow heartbeat.

Bronchiectasis. Dilatation of the bronchi, usually associated with chronic infection.

Bronchiolitis. Inflammation of the bronchioles (tubes that form part of the bronchial tree within the lung), which commonly occurs in infants.

Bronchitis. Inflammation of the bronchi.

Bruit. A rushing sound or murmur within a vessel (French bruit, meaning "noise").

Buccal. Pertaining to the cheek.

Cardiac. Pertaining to the heart.

Cardiac decompensation. Sudden inability of the heart to pump enough blood to meet the metabolic needs of the body.

Cardiac tamponade. Symptoms caused by large accumulation of pericardial fluid: quiet heart, small volume, paradoxical pulse, enlarged liver, and high venous pressure.

Cardiomegaly. Heart enlargement.

Cardiomyopathy. A pathologic condition involving heart muscle.

Carditis. Inflammation of the heart.

Cerebral. Pertaining to the brain, particularly the cerebrum, the largest portion of the brain occupying the whole upper part of the skull cavity.

Cirrhosis. A condition characterized by liver damage.

Coarctation. Narrowing.

Collagen. A component of connective tissue.

Communicable. An infectious disease that can be passed from one person to another.

Congenital. Present at birth.

Conjunctiva. The mucous membrane covering the anterior portion of the globe of the eye.

Consolidation. Process of becoming firm or solid, as in a lung with pneumonia.

Convulsions. Involuntary spasms or muscular contractions, usually referring to epilepsy, originating in the brain.

Costal. Pertaining to the ribs.

Croup. A condition of the larynx seen in children characterized by a harsh, brassy cough and crowing, difficult respiration.

Cyanosis. A bluish tinge of the skin or mucous membranes caused by low arterial blood oxygen.

Decompensation. Failure.

Decubitus. Lying down.

Digitalis. A drug used for treating some forms of heart failure and abnormal rhythm.

Dyspnea. Difficult or labored breathing.

Dystrophy. Abnormal development.

Ectopic beats. Abnormal heartbeats not generated by the normal heart pacemaker.

Edema. Swelling.

Effusion. A pouring out of fluid into a body space.

Emphysema. A condition characterized by overdistention of the air sacs of the lung.

Endocarditis. Inflammation of the membrane (endocardium) lining the chambers of the heart and the valve cusps.

Endocardium. The membrane lining the chambers of the heart and the valve cusps.

Epicanthal fold. A horizontal fold beneath the lower eyelid, characteristic of Down syndrome.

Estrogen. A female sex hormone.

Febrile. Feverish.

Fundal veins. Veins in the retina of the eye visible through the ophthalmoscope.

Gait. Manner of walking.

Glottis. The opening between the free margins of the vocal folds.

Gracile. Long and thin.

Great vessels. The aorta and the pulmonary artery.

Hemoglobin. The red protein in the blood that carries oxygen.

Hemoptysis. The coughing up of blood.

Hepatomegaly. Enlargement of the liver.

Hypertension. Elevated blood pressure.

Hyperventilation. Excessively deep breathing.

Hypoplasia. Underdevelopment.

Hypothyroidism. Underactivity of the thyroid gland.

Hypoxia. Low oxygen content.

In utero. Occurring in the uterus before birth.

Incisura. A slit or notch.

Infarction. A dying of tissue caused by a complete cutoff of blood.

Infundibulum. A funnel-shaped passage or part, usually referring to the area of the right ventricle below the valve.

Intercurrent. Taking place between or during, as an infection that occurs in a patient with cancer.

Ischemia. Local diminution in the blood supply to an organ.

Jaundice. A yellowish discoloration of the skin caused by high levels of bilirubin.

Jugular notch. Depression on the upper surface of the manubrium between the two clavicles.

Lordosis. Forward curvature of the lumbar spine.

Malaise. Sensation of being ill or not well. A vague feeling of bodily discomfort.

Malocclusion. Abnormal closing of the

teeth, usually associated with abnormal development of the jaws.

Mammary. Pertaining to the breast.

Mandible. The jawbone.

Maxillary. Pertaining to the upper jaw.

Micrognathia. Small jaw.

Muscular dystrophy. A genetic disease, beginning in childhood, characterized by early enlargement and later shrinkage of muscles with weakness, a waddling gait, inability to rise from the ground, and progressive helplessness; also called pseudohypertrophic muscular dystrophy.

Myocardiopathy. An abnormality of heart muscle.

Myocarditis. An inflammation of heart muscle.

Myocardium. Heart muscle.

Ori ce. An opening.

Palpebral. Pertaining to the eyelid.

Palpitation. A beating of the heart, often irregular, of which the patient is conscious.

Pansystolic. Occurring throughout systole.

Paroxysm. A spasm or fit.

Pathognomonic. Characteristic of a disease, distinguishing it from other diseases.

Patulous. Expanded or open.

Pericarditis. An inflammation of the pericardium, the membranous sac surrounding the heart.

Petechiae. Small round spots of hemorrhage on the skin or mucous membranes.

Pharynx. The musculomembranous tube situated back of the nose, mouth, and larynx, extending from the base of the skull to the sixth cervical vertebra, where the pharynx joins the esophagus.

Placenta. The organ that attaches the embryo to the uterus by means of the umbilical cord, which supplies it with oxygen and nutrients.

Pleura. The membrane that lines the inside of the chest cavity and covers the lungs.

Polycythemia. A condition characterized by an excess number of red blood cells.

Porcine. Pertaining to a pig.

Postmortem. After death.

Postnatal. After birth.

Precordium. The area of the left side of the chest overlying the heart.

Prenatal. Before birth.

Prognosis. Outlook.

Prone. Lying on the stomach.

Pulmonary. Pertaining to the lungs.

Pulmonary edema. Fluid in the lungs.

Purulent. Pus-filled.

Regurgitation. A backflow.

Resuscitation. The prevention of asphyxial death by artificial respiration.

Shunt. Alternate pathway, bypass, or sidetrack.

Sibling. A brother or sister.

Somnolence. Sleepiness.

Stenosis. Constriction or narrowing.

Stigmata. Marks or signs characteristic of an illness or condition.

Strabismus. Cross-eye.

Subcutaneous. Beneath the skin.

Subluxation. Incomplete dislocation (e.g., of the lens of the eye in Marfan's syndrome).

Supine. Lying on the back (opposite of prone).

Supravalvular. Above a valve.

Syncope. Fainting.

Tachycardia. Rapid heartbeat.

Tachypnea. Rapid breathing.

Thyrotoxicosis. A condition caused by severe overactivity of the thyroid gland.

Toxemia. A condition in which the blood contains poisonous products.

Toxemia of pregnancy. A disease occurring in the second half of pregnancy characterized by acute elevation of blood pressure, protein in the urine, swelling, convulsions, and coma.

Toxicity. Poisonousness.

Transient. Short-lived.

Trimester. A 3-month division of pregnancy (e.g., the first 3 months of pregnancy are the first trimester).

Valsalva maneuver. Forced expiration against a closed glottis.

Vasoconstriction. A narrowing of arteries produced by muscular contraction of their walls.

Vasopressor. A drug that raises arterial pressure.

Venous. Pertaining to the veins.

Viscosity. Quality describing resistance of a liquid to flow (e.g., jelly is more viscous than water).

Index

www.ingramcontent.com/pod-product-compliance
Lightning Source LLC
Chambersburg PA
CBHW051449170526
45166CB00001B/169